Praise for *Tapped in Wellness*

"A must-read for anyone who wants to improve their physical and mental health. Malcolm's unique approach to wellness combines actionable practices and personal experience with concrete science."

—**Giuseppe Federic**, author of *Cooking with Nonna*

"Malcolm's approach to plant-based recipes feels so approachable, nourishing, and fun. I love how he weaves holistic consciousness into his cooking, something we can all learn from! If you are looking to add more plant-forward dishes to your life, *Tapped in Wellness* is the book for you!"

—**Nicole Berrie**, author of *Body Harmony* and founder of Bonberi Mart

"Brilliant read and so helpful for those starting on their wellness journey!"

—**Calum Harris**, cook and author of *The 20-Minute Vegan*

"As a vegan mom and environmental advocate, I'm thrilled to endorse *Tapped in Wellness* for its compassionate approach to nutrition and wellness, echoing the importance of conscious living for ourselves and our children."

—**Ashley Renne Nsonwu**, creator of @HeyAshleyRenne and author of *The Vegan Baby Cookbook and Guide*

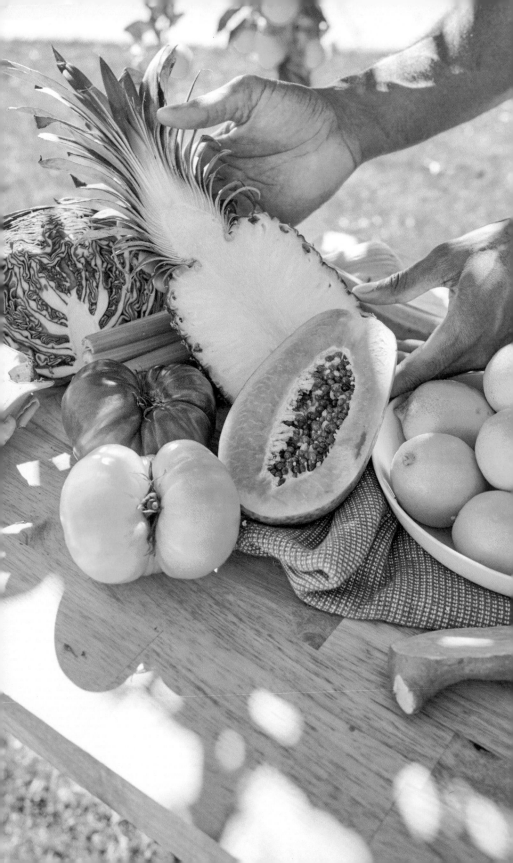

TAPPED IN WELLNESS

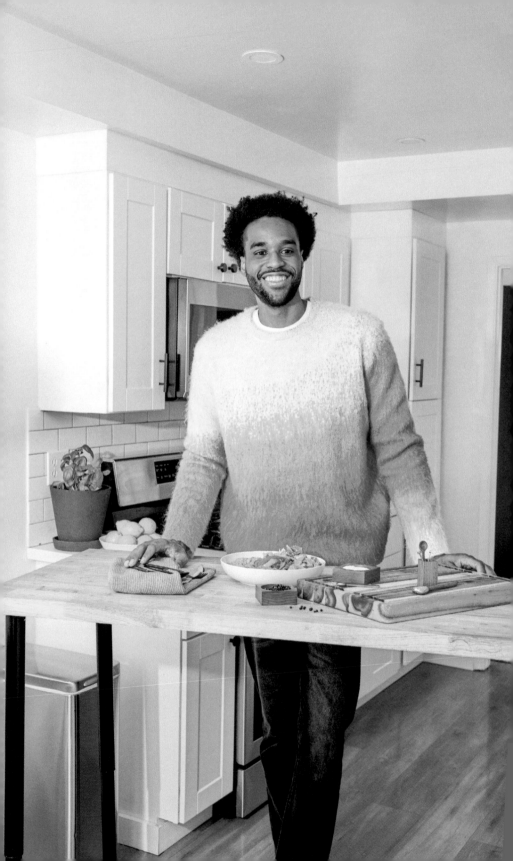

TAPPED IN WELLNESS

Lasting Performance and Health
through Mindful Living and Eating

MALCOLM REGISFORD

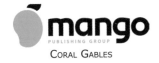

PUBLISHING GROUP

Coral Gables

Cover Design: Elina Diaz
Cover + interior Photography: Talia Dinwiddie
Food stylist: Maddie Eckhoff
Layout & Design: Elina Diaz

For permission requests, please contact the publisher at:
Mango Publishing Group
2850 S Douglas Road, 2nd Floor
Coral Gables, FL 33134 USA
info@mango.bz

For special orders, quantity sales, course adoptions and corporate sales, please email the publisher at sales@mango.bz. For trade and wholesale sales, please contact Ingram Publisher Services at customer.service@ingramcontent.com or +1.800.509.4887.

Tapped in Wellness: Lasting Performance and Health through Mindful Living and Eating

Library of Congress Cataloging-in-Publication number: has been requested
ISBN: (print) 978-1-68481-614-9, (ebook) 978-1-68481-615-6
BISAC category code: SEL016000, SELF-HELP / Personal Growth / Happiness

Printed in the United States of America

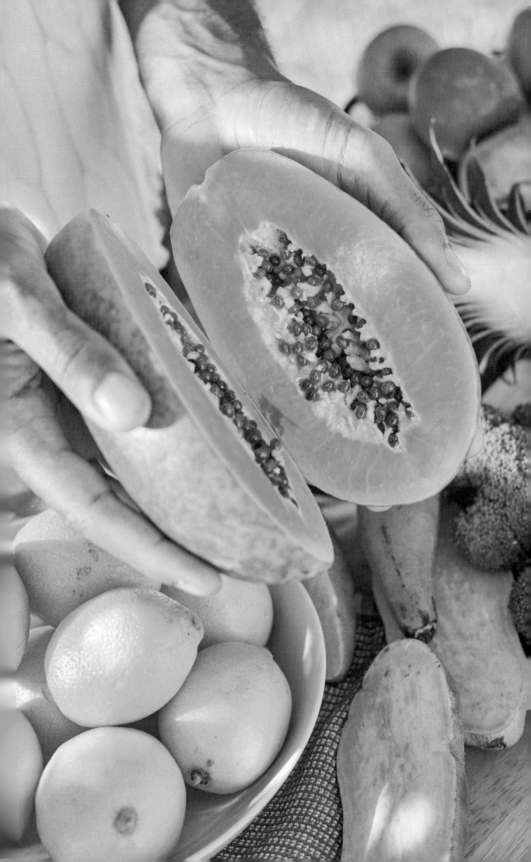

Table of Contents

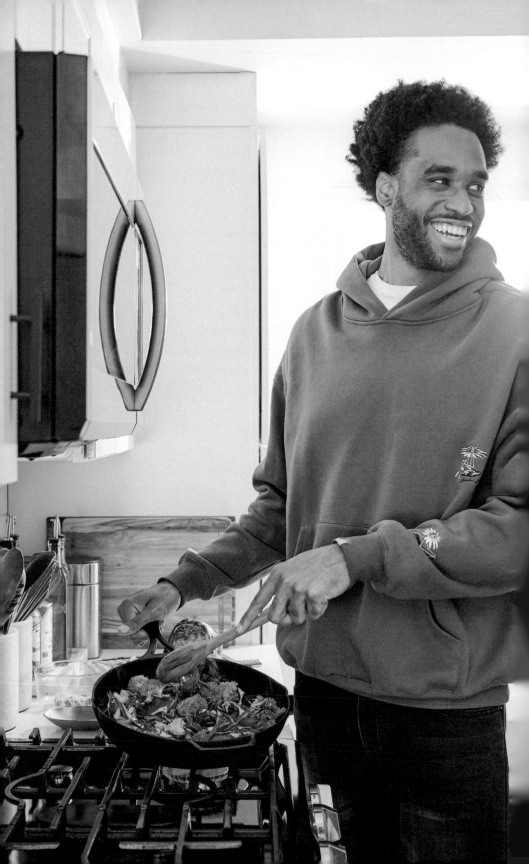

Introduction

Before we start, take in that you're here right now, reading this book, seated in your chair, bed, desk, wherever. No matter what spiritual or religious belief you hold, I feel the power of presence is universal. Taking the time to be rooted in where you are at this moment affords you some opportunities. It enables awareness of so much within yourself and affords you the opportunity to identify anything that might need to be addressed. It also might allow you the chance to give yourself a break or to simply experience the present moment. So, with that in mind, let's do a quick breathing exercise to ground here. It's simple, I promise, and you'll feel good, trust me. Inhale to a count of 4, hold to a count of 7, and exhale to a count of 8. That felt good, right? Let's get started.

The truth is, everything is connected at all times, all at once. Our existence right now is a byproduct of a multitude of factors aligning for us to be here and that stretches back into time way before we could even fathom. We have a symbiotic relationship with the world around us and there's a "call and response," if you will, with everything around us. Anything has the potential to spark a response within us from a song that comes on the radio that reminds you of a fond memory to stubbing your toe first thing in the morning that puts you in a cranky mood the rest of the day. Even something like us being born is a miracle. Our parents were living their individual lives, coming from wherever they come from, and met at a certain time and place in their journey to end up bringing new life into this world, us. They could have made any other decision. They could not have met at all, for all we know, had one or two things been different along the way. That's how incredible it is to take part in the process of creation because we can choose and with everything that can align to aid that process is special. The same goes for any other thing that's ever happened. I'm sure you've had situations where you've contemplated what would have been different had another choice been made, or another factor been introduced, or some other force been exerted. There's a ripple effect from every choice made, and for whatever reason, some ripple led you being here, reading this book. Just take that in for a second.

I've had many of these contemplative moments, for better or for worse. Thinking about everything that could play into certain outcomes could be a useful tool to gauge what you are getting yourself into for the future or could offer a great perspective on the past and how to take lessons from previous experiences. While being a self-proclaimed "overthinker" has provided me with some challenges, over time I've developed a practice that offers me more perspective, more resolve, and true authority over how to interpret the world around me. The practice is built around three pillars of well-being that I feel are foundational elements to true holistic health. These pillars are what I leaned on at pivotal times when I've faced adversity.

I've been an athlete for most of my life, dedicating hours upon hours to become the best version of myself I could envision. The sport I had the most affinity for, as well as ability, was basketball. Over time I earned a Division 1 scholarship and accomplished one of my lifetime goals. The true adversity came into play the summer before my junior year when I was experiencing some lingering soreness in my ankle. This turned out to be bone spurs and worn-down cartilage and required surgery to correct, sidelining me for months of recovery. Upon returning to campus that fall my ankle still hadn't healed as much as I'd hoped, delaying my return to action with the upcoming season weeks away at this point. Eventually, I decided to return to play, but I still wasn't where I wanted to be physically. At this time, I was also seeing my integral role on the team change in real time to a secondary one due to my impaired physical condition—something I hadn't experienced before. Add to it the diminishing support from those I'd entrusted my development with up to this point within the program, being away from home and family across the country, having to shoulder the responsibilities of a high-performing educational institution and trying to grapple with my identity as an athlete for the first time. All of this left me on an island to deal with my recovery.

In a time when I felt the odds were stacked against me, I had no choice but to look within. I already felt beside myself having my identity as an athlete challenged so greatly. For anyone, whether you are or have been an athlete or not, I'm sure you can relate to a time when something you were so heavily identified with, in this case my body's ability to perform, was challenged or taken away. This turned the tide for me in so many ways. I started to audit my life in a way, analyzing everything I was taking in and surrounded myself with to determine if it served me or not. I was building, without knowing it at the time, the pillars of health that would help lead me to a better version of myself.

It started with the first pillar of mental/spiritual health, taking account of my thoughts, the narratives I was telling myself, becoming aware of patterns I wanted to change, what I was consuming and differentiating between what I feel and what's real. The second pillar came into play with physical health, building a mind-body connection through a healthier relationship with movement, understanding what makes me feel good instead of following ideologies blindly and orienting my physical environment to help serve what I wanted to achieve. The third pillar of nutritional wellness, particularly whole-food plant-based eating, was one of the more transformative aspects of the process by way of reframing my idea of food and the power it holds to heal. Seeing that change in real-time once I switched from what I thought was a trial period to what became a lifestyle choice, just to get me back to playing, left a big impression on me.

With as many factors as there are in the world, it could seem like we have no control at all, like things are random or "just happen," especially when it comes to things that are external to us. For the most part, this is true. But while there is plenty we can't control, I've found that the realm of influence we have over our environment, personal circumstances, relationships, minds, and bodies leaves important impressions. Like I said, *everything* is connected. If there's anything I'd want you to take away from this, it's that you do have the power to change your reality. You're already doing it daily, just in smaller ways. From the dish you choose for dinner to the show you want to watch, this is all information for your body and mind that creates a certain response. The key is identifying what information evokes what response and determining if you like it, if it contributes to what you want to feel, do, or accomplish.

In this book, I aim to share my experience through these pillars as well as offer some of the tools I've learned, adapted, and implemented in my life, in hopes that it inspires you to do some of the same in yours. This isn't a one-size-fits-all method by any means. The beauty of holistic health is that it is individual and customizable. The things you end up doing may look like what I offer here or different. The real goal is taking the steps toward what this looks like for you and tapping into more what you know yourself to be, taking the power back over health and well-being and feeling like the best version of yourself along the way.

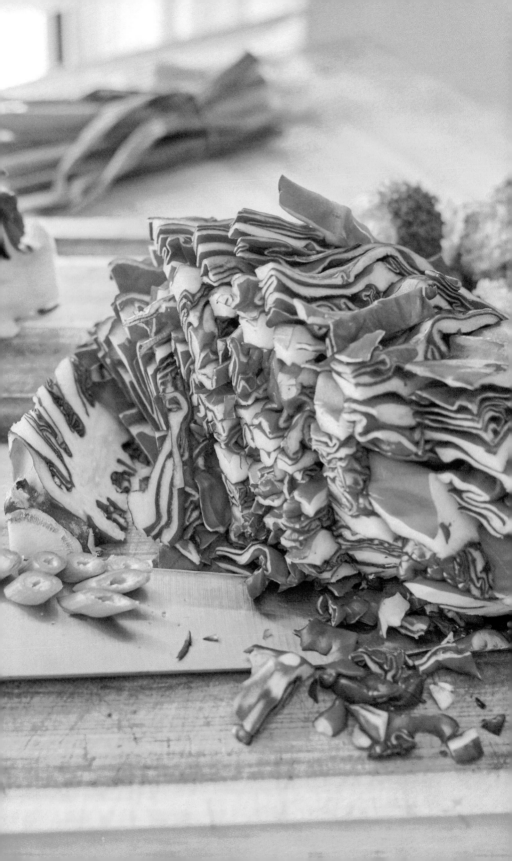

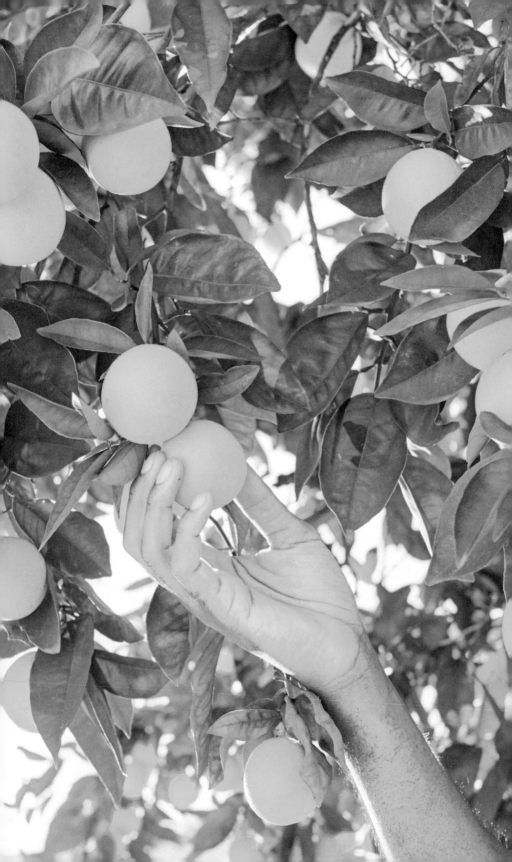

MENTAL + SPIRITUAL WELLNESS:

TAKING STOCK OF YOUR PERSONAL HIGHLIGHT REEL

Whether you've ever stepped onto any field of competition like a basketball court or soccer pitch or been part of any team competing for a trophy, you're an athlete. But instead of competing within a designated arena with spectators and referees, you're playing the sport of life. In the sport of life, you're your own trainer, your own coach, your own teammate, your own biggest fan, and sometimes, worst critic. Unlike many sports where you have ample time to train and build skills, strength, and conditioning as well as forge a game plan based on an opponent, there's no way to prepare for what life has in store. There's no scouting report on life circumstances, nothing to forecast how the things we want to happen will pan out, who will be our romantic partner, when or where the next work opportunity will come from and all this anticipation can lead to stress and anxiety if we're not careful.

Trying to control all these things is where we go wrong as a society and culture at large. Independent of any belief, philosophy, or religion you hold, despite any practice you implement, the idea that the onus is all on us as an individual to build the life we want through willpower alone is honestly overwhelming and ultimately not true. All the clips of so-called business gurus will have you thinking it all has to be difficult and that you have to exert so much energy before anything can be done. I'll tell you from experience that not everything has to come from hardship. You're not alone in this journey and your ability as a creator is more powerful than you might give it credit for.

At times it can certainly feel as if you are alone on a path toward something and yes, as an individual you are responsible for setting things into motion, taking action with clear intention, and following through on those intentions, but that is only one piece of the puzzle. Elements, people, circumstances, opportunities, miracles can all present themselves along the way to contribute to your vision. The biggest responsibility you have is to be aware enough to notice them, see you are supported, and keep moving.

There is one tool you can use to take yourself to the next level and equip yourself for the sport of life and that's becoming more aware of your highlight reel. A highlight reel is the tape you watch on repeat and rehearse to get ready to face an opponent. This is key to how the game plays out in the end. It's important that this reel is thorough, comprehensive, and tailored to the information that will help you come out on top. In the sport of life, the highlight reel I'm referring to is the one that runs in your mind and can determine your mental, emotional, and spiritual health in response to what gets thrown at you. In other words, the difference between a win and a loss, both of which are valuable.

A win is a confirmation that what you're doing is working; it's a sign you're on the right path and can continue to use the tools you've amassed to move forward. A loss, although commonly held with a negative connotation has great value in that it shows what isn't working, what might need improvement, and how to adjust. In other words, giving you more information on how to win! Let's be honest— the losses never feel good. I'll be the first to say it: losing sucks. It can be discouraging, it can be frustrating but coming out on the other side of the emotional experience, you always know what lesson, improvement, or adjustment you can extract to perform better on the next opportunity, even if it takes some time.

Your highlight reel is the composition of what you consume mentally and how you relate those thoughts, ideas, and narratives back to yourself through repetition, or "reps" for short. And just like you can improve your jump shot or develop more strength at the gym with reps, the same goes for the way you use one of your most important muscles, the mind. There is a lot that makes up this muscle; it's the stories you believe about who you are in relation to the world, the things you've been told about yourself, and what you learned about what's true or false, right or wrong. Whether it's come from a certain upbringing or has developed over time with experience, your highlight reel is your only responsibility to manage. Keeping the narratives you repeat and rehearse in check and aligned with what you want to accomplish makes a difference in how you respond under the arena lights. And as much as the sport of life has no playbook, the approach of a champion is key to victory.

Conscious Consumption

What comes to mind when you hear the word *consume*? The biggest associations you probably have with this word are likely related to food consumption, even media or business, as it pertains to how companies market to "consumers." Whatever your first thought was, consuming is all you do. It happens on many levels from consuming food to live and nourish yourself to the relationships you have with people and their effect on your state of being to the social media scrolling, books being read, TV and movies being watched or any other form of entertainment you take in daily. All of this input leaves an impression whether you are aware of it or not. The conscious mind can take in information and, with effort and repetition, it can retain it.

The subconscious mind is like a camera that's always rolling, capturing everything and forming a psychological makeup that you then have the choice to accept. Some people never make this decision and are subject to the aftermath of a mass of ideas that don't serve them and that don't contribute to their highest self. This is why it is so important to be aware of what you consume outside of what foods you eat. The brain is a sponge and it's your job to ensure that it absorbs what you want.

We are extremely impressionable beings, more than we give credit to. Our minds are amalgamations of things we've learned, been exposed to, and internalized as truth. As time goes on, we become more hardwired in our habits, patterns, and processes, and the information we have taken in sets in deeper, but context is everything. All it takes is a reframe of a few elements around you, add in some repetition, and it can completely shift what you might think, feel, or do in any situation.

When I was playing college basketball and was faced with injury and a lack of emotional support, I felt as if I was on an island alone and everything that got thrown at me took a lot out of me. I was dealing with these things from a reactive frame of mind. It'd become apparent that the ideas I had consumed up to this point no longer served me as

I was thrust into a new context from which to operate. It was sort of a sink-or-swim moment now that I look back on it. I had consumed and internalized the idea that I'd recover from my injury and everything around me would return to normal on my terms—my role on the team, the dynamics with my teammates and coaches, my physical state—but none of that presented itself to me, so my reality was met with resistance.

This resistance led to more negative thoughts that framed me as a victim in the situation and made me feel powerless and like the only source of validation would come from those external to me. During this time, because I was focused so much on getting fed from the external world and saw that I wasn't getting the response I wanted, I had to turn my attention inward. To this day I can't tell you what made me want to go this route, given that I was so wrapped up in what I wanted other people, outside circumstances, and forces to do for me. I don't know what made me choose this path as opposed to another because there were times I wanted to bow out, leave school, quit basketball, the whole nine, because I was so strongly identified with my role as an athlete. With the perspective I have now, I know it might have been easy to quit but that would have sent me down a rabbit hole of regret and self-defeating thoughts. All I knew was one day I wanted to stop feeling powerless, so I decided to walk toward taking that power back.

I knew something had to change and I thought if the environment or people around me weren't going to give me what I needed, I had to give it to myself. It started with what I was taking in, believing, and internalizing. It started with social media. I noticed the accounts I was following weren't contributing anything positive to my life. I'd doom scroll for hours, not absorbing anything useful and would just be mindlessly passing the time. I realized this was a coping mechanism to numb my brain after feeling so drained from fighting against all these external factors I'd set against myself.

What sparked the shift was a friend's Instagram page. He played college basketball but would post more about his health and wellness along with spirituality-based, self-development content, just as a means of expressing himself. I noticed when I saw his posts or stories, they'd resonate. Most of them pertained to expanding your awareness and becoming more in tune with your mind and emotions to become a fuller being, and I began to take an interest in his posts more, looking forward to what idea he would present next. This is when I started to become introduced to the idea that shifting the focus to yourself could be beneficial and how, if we're not careful, the way we rely on the outside world to validate us, uplift us, or give us permission to be who we want can lead to a large amount of disappointment and lay the groundwork for manipulation of emotions and thoughts, ultimately drawing us away from our truest self. This also taught me that you never know who is watching and what is normal or mundane for you could spark something profound in another person. That's what my friend's posts did for me, along with others who presented themselves on this path. So keep being you because you never know who you might be influencing.

Once these ideas landed, it was impossible to unsee. I became so sensitive to what information, perspectives, and entertainment I wanted to take in. If it didn't make me feel good or contribute to the vision I had for myself moving forward, it had to go. I performed somewhat of an audit on my media consumption, cutting down who I was following and replacing them with people and accounts that made me feel aligned and empowered. The music I listened to became more attuned to affirmative lyrics and messaging. Certain TV shows and movies inspired me to continue on the path I was carving out for myself. These all had a major role in revitalizing my mental health and setting me on a new trajectory that impacted how I trained physically and what I consumed nutritionally shortly after. But we'll get to that later.

I'd encourage you to consider what you consume daily outside of what you eat and how it might be affecting you for better or worse with these three tips to start:

Perform a Media Audit

Our minds are most impressionable when we're in a relaxed state and we most often consume media when we're relaxed. Having our guard down after a long day and then watching depressing news stories or scrolling social media to see posts of people telling you you're doing life wrong is a recipe for a constant undercurrent of stress and anxiety about the world and our place in it in comparison to others. I know not everyone does this and not every account you follow or show you watch is negative, but nonetheless it would be wise to consider the things you absorb in your relaxed state because they're much more likely to leave an impression, and these impressions are the basis for thought patterns that could help or harm you.

If It Doesn't Feel Good, It's Got to Go

This is the simplest one. If what you're consuming makes you feel on edge, annoyed, or drained, let it go. It's not worth your time and energy to be worried about what you expose yourself to. There should be an agreement within yourself that you know you'll have your own back as far as prioritizing feeling good. Most of the time we look for other people or other things to give this to us or feel it has to be earned or is contingent upon some other entity, but this doesn't have to be the case. We're risking our well-being if we depend solely on external forces for gratification. Claim feeling good and doing things because you want to. How many accounts or people do you follow on social media that you don't care about? How many posts do you wish you hadn't seen? What shows and movies are you sitting through mindlessly just to pass the time? Align your means of consumption to feed you so you feel satisfied.

See What You Want to Be

In addition to assessing and eliminating what doesn't feel good, you have to add back in what does. When I began shifting my media consumption, I added in all the social accounts, movies, TV, and music that embodied what I wanted to see and inspired me. It can be the smallest adjustments too. This doesn't mean you have to do an overhaul on everything you've ever watched but tuning in more to learn what works for you and what doesn't could make a big difference over time.

I learned almost everything I know now about cooking, transitioning to being plant-based as a high-performing athlete, and spirituality from someone that I added to my social feeds and TV screens as a means to reprogram the mindless activity I was engaged in before and didn't allow me to change unhealthy patterns. Treat yourself like an experiment and see if you can rewire the patterns that have built up that don't serve you by giving yourself some positive propaganda, if you will, in the form of people, places, and things that inspire you and feed you every time you log on.

The Power of Meditation

The data is already in on this and luckily practices like mindfulness and meditation are having a mainstream moment, so the idea isn't as foreign or "woo-woo" as it once was. It's no secret this is something that can be beneficial but if you were ever on the fence about starting or were skeptical about how it might work for you, hopefully this section could offer some more context for you to decide to try.

I heard an analogy on *Headspace Guide to Meditation* on Netflix (a great introduction to meditation and how to get started) and it described meditation as sitting on the side of a road and watching cars pass.

Your goal is to sit and watch the passing cars on the road. The road represents your mind and the passing cars represent your thoughts. Again, the goal is to observe the cars, but sometimes you get anxious by the speed of the cars or how many cars are on the road. Sometimes you might even chase after a few or run out in the middle of the road to try and stop them altogether. But this only creates more frustration and restlessness within the practice. You may forget the idea is to observe, let them pass, and aim to change your perspective on them rather than alter them. This changed the way I viewed meditation.

Meditation is a practice that offers a host of benefits, from stress reduction to enhanced mental clarity and more. It's also a truly universal practice as it can be implemented regardless of your beliefs. It's been used across cultures spanning mass amounts of time. It allows you to hit pause on the running tape you have in your head and offers moments of solace from the day ahead of you, relief from the events that have passed, and presence in the moment in front of you.

Meditating can impact your well-being on all levels, from mental and physical to spiritual. No matter what activity you partake in daily, they all have an effect on these three areas and they all have a different entry point. One example is doing a physical activity like working out which physically exerts the body but releases endorphins that link to the mental entry point and boosts our emotional state, which can set you up for the rest of your day on a positive note.

I like to think of our state of being as operating from series of starting points; if you wake up in the morning and instantly receive bad news that affects you negatively, that might put you at a lower set point vibrationally to start your day and you might have to do more work to get yourself back up to a vibrational state that you want to be in. Maybe listen to some good music, talk to a loved one, or do something like a short meditation to re-center. When your vibrational set point is on the lower end, you operate from that and it might mean you're more irritable. Small things that usually don't bother you now do, and you're resisting your daily circumstances and being overall a lesser version of yourself. This also takes you out of alignment with what you might want to accomplish for that day and, if sustained over a long time, your life.

You can only attract what you're in alignment with. For example, if I want to try a new vegan restaurant but instead, when I go out I go to a place I already know because I'm afraid I won't like this new place or I don't want to go alone and set up these roadblocks for myself, it makes it impossible for me to attract new experiences.

The same goes the other way. If to start your day you received some good news, didn't have to be in traffic on your daily commute, or had a good meal, odds are that set point would be much higher. Things would feel much more in flow; you're not as bothered about the small things, you can work toward more solutions, and it's an overall easier day. Think about how good you feel once you've completed a workout and how maybe everything that happens throughout the course of the day might not affect you as negatively because you got that mental and physical boost earlier in the day because emotionally and spiritually you're at a higher set point. But if you're subject to a lot of stress throughout the day and are mentally at odds with what you are dealing with on a regular basis, the mental entry point has a link to a physiological response of stress within the nervous system. This could trigger things like higher blood pressure and raised cortisol and adrenaline levels. Too much of this can break down the body and its functions over time and lower your vibrational set point on the spiritual front.

By keeping the body in "survival mode," so to speak, you don't give it a chance to allot any energy or resources to the areas that are linked to replenishing, regenerating, and recovering because everything internally says that the body is in danger. It will bypass healing or rest to keep all assets in the areas of producing stress hormones to aid the perpetual state of "danger" that the body feels you're in. Even your natural mental and physical responses can be hijacked without awareness of what triggers them and without the tools to self-regulate when needed. This can cascade into a habitual imprint that can have you participating in behavioral patterns that don't serve you.

Meditation can be one of the tools to bring you back to where you need to be.

Meditation is like hitting the refresh button on a web page that's been buffering for way too long. It can refresh all these entry points all at once and recalibrate them so you can run more efficiently. Physically, it puts you in a grounded and relaxed state, releasing all tension in the body and breathing consciously to foster a rest response in the brain, which leads to the mental entry point. Managing your breathing or even just being physically relaxed tells the brain it's okay to rest and therefore produces neurochemicals like GABA, the neurotransmitter responsible for calming the brain and which activates in the parasympathetic nervous system. A calmer and relaxed mental/physical state means a cleaner slate to work from, which allows for the inner spiritual and vibrational processes to take place. The thoughts that wouldn't stop racing seem less overwhelming now and the things you were worried about have melted away and you have more perspective on how to move forward.

Think of your mind before meditation as a messy house—things are scattered everywhere, loads of clutter, unorganized, and you don't know where things are or how to process the space you're in. And imagine you want to throw a party and have people over in this house; it'd be impossible. To have new people and energy in the house while the initial mess hasn't been dealt with or cleared away would only add more stress to trying to host this event that could bring positivity.

So, think of a meditation as a deep cleaning of your house, a reorganization so that the new people you invite over can feel comfortable and enjoy the space. But how do you do this? Is it just breathing? Do you have to sit in silence for hours until you reach enlightenment? The answer is yes and no. Meditation can take many forms and luckily that means more people can participate and customize the experience so they can get the most out of it. If that means taking five minutes to sit without your phone or any outside stimulation, that could work. If you want to incorporate box breathing or the Wim Hof method, that works too. Give yourself time to tap into something creative or fall into an activity you enjoy for a while. There are a million roads that lead to the same destination and the journey there is just as rewarding.

The stereotypical idea people have of meditation is that you have to sit with your legs crossed, humming and moaning while you turn your brain off. The truth is there is no right way to mediate and that image couldn't be further from what it is. Yes, that is a form of meditation, but that doesn't mean you have to do it like that to get the benefits from it. There are elements of the practice you can develop and integrate wherever you are at any stage in your journey, and you can tailor it so you get the most of what you're looking for.

First, meditation is about feeling comfortable, getting yourself into a safe space physically and feeling like you can let go, whether this is in your bedroom, car, or workspace. The goal is to anchor into your physical body so you can move within. This also doesn't have to happen one way, such as sitting down, eyes closed, and zoning out. Meditation can come through many active forms. How many times have you been working on something you're passionate about—making a piece of art, cooking a meal, listening to great music, having a great workout at the gym, or reading a good book—and felt like everything else has melted away? And all that is, is that moment, that activity, that sensation, that flow state. You've just experienced a form of meditation. Meditation can be an active thing and whether you've sat for hours chanting mantras or taking five minutes to sit and breathe mindfully, you have the power to access a greater state of clarity and then move forward in the rest of your day.

Another aspect I hear people complain about a lot when trying to get into meditation is "my mind keeps racing" or "I couldn't stop thinking so I gave up." That isn't the point of such a practice. It's almost impossible to stop all thoughts from forming and presenting themselves in our minds at any point because that's what it is made to do. Our brain's function is to conceptualize, calculate, and think, and we need that to survive. It's clearly served our species well because we've survived this long. It's not bad that you can't turn this off. On the flip side, this tool has been hijacked by our society and culture through an information and stimulus overload. This makes us process information about so many things at once through sheer exposure. Everything has to be analyzed; everything has to be absorbed. Think about how many ads you see throughout the day or how many headlines online are reaching for your attention or how many times your phone screen lights up with notifications and buzzes, causing micro dopamine spikes throughout the day. In a way, we're micro-dosing these stress signals from having to process so much. I can see how it'd be harder to feel grounded during a session.

But even with that, the approach to starting a meditation practice is key because you can start even if you feel you're someone who can't turn your brain off. No matter how long you've been meditating, you'll find some thoughts you can't turn off with a switch, but the beauty is that with time you can sit with your thoughts and not be overwhelmed by them. You'll observe them from a somewhat neutral point of view. It's like zooming out on a bunch of information and viewing it more as a spectator.

Meditation is also about making space in the mind, decluttering the things we don't need and allowing the new to come in. If you sit with a thought long enough, you might find it doesn't need as much energy as you're giving it. It might seem unimportant. Usually thoughts feel more overwhelming because they are compounded by many other thoughts of the same level rushing through at the same time, and often, each thought isn't so severe. It's like a game of *Whac-A-Mole*. The game is intense because all the moles pop up randomly in a short amount of time, but if it were only one mole popping up, you'd know exactly how to handle it and it'd be less stressful. Taking time to sit with all the thoughts that pop up over a session and view them objectively, nonjudgmentally, and without attaching a story to them is a huge tool in your kit that affords you more bandwidth to field more throughout the day.

In addition to being aware of what you consume, meditation is a great tool to regulate your personal highlight reel and ensure it is up to par for you to perform at your best. You deserve to be at your best. Here are my top tips for starting and maintaining a meditation practice:

Start with Five Minutes

Everyone has five minutes at some point in their day. Take these minutes to first put your phone down, turn on Do Not Disturb, turn off any screens, and get in a comfortable position. You could turn on calming music or background noise, close your eyes, and pay attention to your breathing. Feel your belly going in and out, feel the cool air enter your nostrils as you breathe in, and fall into a deeper state of relaxation as you exhale. Just start here. Do not be concerned with whether you're doing it right or not because there is no right or wrong here. Your thoughts might be racing, you may feel anxious about starting, but as you put more time in, the thoughts become less pronounced and you'll shift your focus inward. Afterward, you'll feel better. Giving yourself a moment to pause has more of an effect than you might realize, even if it's only for five minutes.

Set Your Intention

Another reason why meditation practice doesn't stick for people is because they don't know why they're doing it. They hear it is good for you or hop on because it's trendy, but after they try it a few times, they don't know what they're looking for and end up falling off. Something that anchors you in any practice is finding the why in it (foreshadowing much?). Aside from a general motivation to get into the practice, it helps to set an intention for each session. Questions you could ask yourself would be: why am I meditating right now? Is it to calm nerves? Is it to release anger? Is it simply to feel more grounded? Is it to express gratitude? Distinguishing the aim of your practice sets the tone for you to key in on specific

emotions, thought patterns, or behaviors you feel would benefit you on the other side of the session.

This also goes back to those set points I mentioned before. Take notice of where you are on that scale throughout the day. Take notice of what might be contributing to your state of being, whether it's good or bad, so when you take the time to meditate, you know what you're aiming to build upon.

Stay Consistent

You can't expect to get better or feel more comfortable with anything if you don't put the time in and get those reps. The same applies to meditation. You might not feel the clarity or peace you're looking for right off the bat, especially if you haven't tried it before, so you have to give it a real shot before you decide definitively that it's not for you, just like with any other skill or habit you want to build. I'm proposing you make a commitment to twenty-one days. That's three weeks to see if this is something that could benefit you. Work it into your routine, whether it's first thing in the morning or right before you go to bed but give yourself the time to dedicate to you and the practice. Twenty-one days, five to ten minutes a day, is the goal. Are you up for it?

Finding Your "Why"

Why do we do anything we do? There's a reason you get up every day and go to work or school, dedicate time to a passion of yours, or spend time with loved ones. You do those things because they offer you something that you feel positively contributes to your life in some way. Though you may not consciously be thinking about all the reasons why you do all that you do, the underlying motivation remains. It's the connection to that motivation that allows you to keep doing those things, even in difficult times. This is why finding your why to lean on when you're on a path of self-discovery is crucial. Taking on this type of journey is no easy feat. First, give yourself credit for taking the first step in that direction. Your why is what guides you. It's what shapes your gut instinct and nudges you toward the next steps in actualizing your desires.

Overall, this is a simple concept, but there are levels to it. Of course, finding out why you want to do something is simple because you have the end result in mind, but it's also helpful to consider where the why comes from. What this means is delving into the motivation behind the motivation. Let's say your goal is to have one million followers on social media. Do you want those followers because you feel you have something to offer an audience? Is it coming from a place of insecurity? Do you want to entertain? Do you want to troll? This all matters. Taking time to understand what you want to get out of a certain endeavor is one thing but considering what it might take to get there and how you want to go about it is another.

I like to think about the why in the context of a superhero movie. There's the hero and villain. Both have their whys. If you were to ask these characters what they want, they'd probably say similar things— how they want a better world, equality, or justice for a cause they believe in. But how they plan to go about that is the bigger question. The villain might want to shift a power structure or leverage people's well-being to get to this vision, while the hero wants to keep things as they are and protect people so they can make their own decisions. Both are in the process of creation and both are operating from their why. Watching these movies showed me, especially as I've gotten older, that the process of creation is literal. Both characters are doing what they set out to do and taking steps toward their goal. Regardless of the means, they are creating from their why but in different ways. Who is to say one is right or wrong?

There are levels to knowing your why. But I'll reel it back in to think about this in the context of taking steps toward a new lifestyle change or goal. Knowing you want to, for example, work out more to compete in a bodybuilding contest as opposed to feeling better in your body. There are two different approaches and two different means. It's the same why of wanting to work out more but the underlying, more nuanced goal within the why determines a different outcome and process. So, I'd encourage you to find your why but then look deeper and ask where it's coming from. Is it from a place of self-love, insecurity, empowerment, or fear? Whichever it is, know it and decide if the initial intention needs to be adjusted to fit what you want to accomplish because there are many ways to get to the same place, but it's about what you're willing to do to get there that can be the determining factor in creating a new reality.

It would seem by society's standards that there is always something we could be doing better. There's always another fitness trend that's sure to get you the body of your dreams or another diet you should be using to fix every health problem there ever was or a productivity tip that is almost guaranteed to make you a millionaire. These ideas are pushed on us every day and at the same time we're made to feel we've been doing life wrong the whole time. While it is great to continue to look for ways to improve, evolve, and grow, this motivation needs to come from within—or at the least start there.

You need to know why you're doing what you're doing. You need to know why you feel it will contribute positively to your life and why you feel it's worth it to put in the effort to get you there. Otherwise you'll feel jerked in every direction by what the external world is telling you is the "right" thing to do. Leave it up to the outside world and you'll never be satisfied. External motivation or influence is part of the process and is useful if applied correctly to fuel your intrinsic why and in some cases expand your mind to what else is available or possible. The other side of that coin is the external as a driving force for comparison which can veer you off your intended path. There's so much being pushed on us and so many people find success using different methods. It's impossible to compare such circumstances to yours as some sort of measuring stick or to adopt everything that claims to be a quick fix. I also know this can be difficult.

As humans we're prone to these emotions as we're a tribal and communal species, so naturally the experiences of others will leave an impression on us. We also are exposed to so much these days with the expansion of social media. The accessibility we have to others' lives is something no generation has had to face before and it's not always as good as we might think. By no means is our growth in access to information inherently bad. It's great to stay connected to who we care about, but there's a blurred line between a casual life update or an entertaining video on our feed and an overload of info from hundreds of peers' day-to-day activities, most of which aren't relevant to your activities but carry weight in the sense of how your life might measure up to theirs.

Outside influences can make our why murky at times and get in the way of what we set out to do simply because we saw someone do it another way. It's always great to be introduced to new information but a constant influx of it can interfere with the original intention. From the view of the outside world, there will always be something else to do and a way to do it better than it was done before. Think about how many versions of the iPhone have come out. Why do we need a new phone every year? The models don't change that much from year to year and aside from a few new minor modifications, you'll essentially have the same phone as last year. Most often, additions like this don't add to the quality of your life in any significant way, but we don't take enough time to think about how necessary it is to jump into something just because someone or something tells us to.

The system is designed to keep a perpetual state of desire flowing so that those who aimlessly desire will fall into the new thing. These things that are being sold—and I don't just mean material goods but ideologies, habits, and lifestyle practices—are products too, just as much as that new iPhone. Except with these other products you don't pay with money; you pay with your peace of mind and self-assurance. Now, I'm not telling you not to get a new phone if that's what you feel you need. I am telling you that you should know why you want a new phone, why you want to make a lifestyle change, or why you want to take on a new habit or learn a new skill. Knowing why solidifies your power in the exchange and ensures you'll get the most out of what you decide to embark on.

Out of the who, what, where, when, why, and how, the why is the most important part of the process of creation and the part you're most responsible for. No one can cast out your intention or know what you want more than you. A ship can't set sail and a plane can't take flight without knowing its direction, even if it knows where it wants to end up. While it's the most important part of the process, it's also the most fun because you get to paint whatever picture you want for yourself and no one can tell you otherwise. It galvanizes your internal motivation and pushes you toward aligned action. The rest of the elements, like who will be involved, when it will happen, and how it will happen, are not up to you and are largely out of your control.

Even with a solid plan, there is no way to forecast what is in store in totality. Elements may come into play that haven't been considered yet because you don't know what you don't know. If you have a strong connection to the why and allow that to be your guide, the rest aligns in relation to it. Remember what I said about setting your intentions in the last section? Knowing your why is much like that. Even not knowing these other factors puts you on a path that unfolds as you move through it in real-time. It also reveals surprises along the way.

The motivation behind why you want to do anything new will also be what anchors you in the process, even if it is something you don't enjoy. People go to jobs they don't enjoy every day, but they know why they do. At the least it's to survive and provide for themselves or their families, and sometimes that's all it takes. Or you might not like your household chores, but you know why you do them—to have a clean and tidy living space, which enhances your quality of life. The connection to motivation is paramount in creating what you want because our desires change, priorities shift, and needs fluctuate. It's a fluid experience regarding what we want at a given time but knowing your why gives you the buoyancy to ride those waves.

The why is what stakes your claim in any endeavor and gives you the power to direct your energy toward your intention. I know in my experience when I was facing my injury and identity crisis as an athlete, going inward and realizing that my desires, priorities, and needs had all been turned upside down forced me to recalibrate and find a new why, a new anchor. I also didn't consciously set out to make this as pronounced as I'm making it to you now, but all I knew at the time was a feeling that called me to find solutions and align myself with what I wanted to experience, which at that time was feeling like myself in my body and mind again.

Experiencing an injury that wasn't healing as expected plus dealing with my identity as an athlete challenged for the first time ever in that way and feeling like I was disconnected from myself pushed me to find the why that is still my why today: to be well, healthy, self-sufficient, and hold dominion over how I experience my thoughts and body and everything in between. I knew I didn't want anyone or any circumstance but me to have control over that.

If we keep looking outward for the validation we seek for ourselves, we won't get it. Or if we do, it will be fleeting and therefore we'll always be chasing something external. While it's good to have healthy outlets where we can relinquish the need to have control or power over certain life elements and rely on some outside help, ultimately that acceptance has to come from you. So don't think that your why has to be this fully fleshed out master plan for it to yield results but rather tap into the feelings you have about what you're envisioning. Listen to the voice that's deep within and trust that you'll be okay along the way.

If you don't feel connected to your why or you want to delve deeper into the why you already have, here are three questions you can ask yourself to lend more clarity to your search:

What Is the Intended Goal?

It's hard to know what you can do about something if you don't know what you're aiming for. Asking what the intended goal is takes you to the result and begins to set forth a line of possibilities that you can act on in the moment or in the near future. As important as it is to know why you want to do something, knowing what you want to do will spring you into action and be an additional driving force to discover more.

How Will You Feel When You Get This?

As well as knowing what you want to do, it is vital to have this envisioned reality aligned with a feeling. Our feelings set the charge for that experience. Think about how you feel when you think about a night out with friends as opposed to doing taxes. Both have different emotional charges and you approach those two experiences with different mindsets. When on the path to actualizing your vision, using your emotions to put you in a state of openness and receptivity can speed up the process because you're in flow vibrationally. Even something tedious like taxes can be framed in a light that has you feeling as exuberant as if you were going out with your friends. So think about how it would feel to receive or accomplish your goal and use that feeling to fuel your efforts.

What Do You Feel Called to Do about This Right Now?

This is an underrated one because if you think about it, there is always *something* to be done. Whether that something will lead to where you want, we don't always know. But instead of aimlessly taking on tasks or exerting yourself in the name of being "productive," tune into what you feel *inspired* to do in the moment. I use the word *inspired* carefully because the idea of inspiration is akin to a sense of feeling taken over by motivation to get something done. While this feeling occurs, if we rely solely on that to move things along, our efforts will be few and far between. Set up a structure or dedicate time to these efforts so you can make your action habitual.

There is always something to be doing but it's key to tune in and feel into what you could do that would feel good and contribute to the goal. The other side is aimless action in the name of the goal but has no real directive. Whenever I feel caught about what to do, I first think about whether the efforts feel aligned emotionally and then frame the action I take through what feels best. Sometimes that means taking a break and doing nothing. Think about what this means for you and how your actions are best needed at a certain point. This balance reminds me of a Denzel Washington quote that embodies the essence of this approach: "Just because you're doing a lot more, doesn't mean you're getting a lot more done...don't confuse movement with progress, you could run in place all day and never get anywhere."

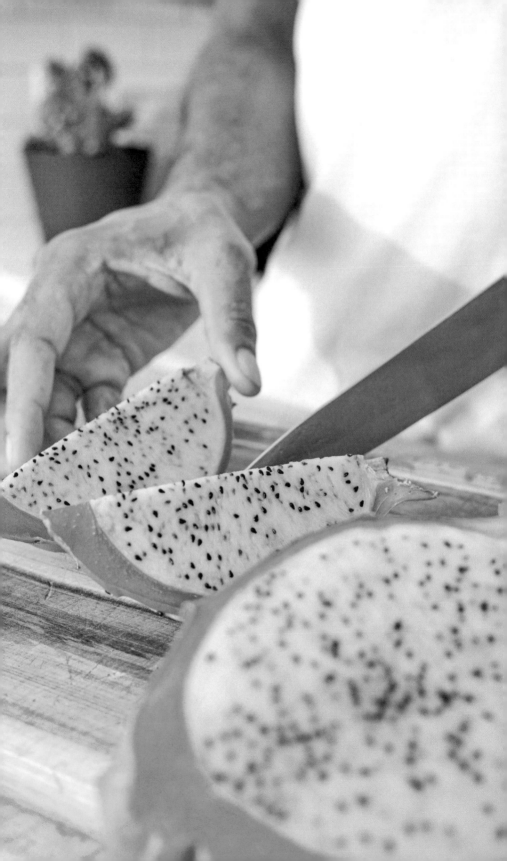

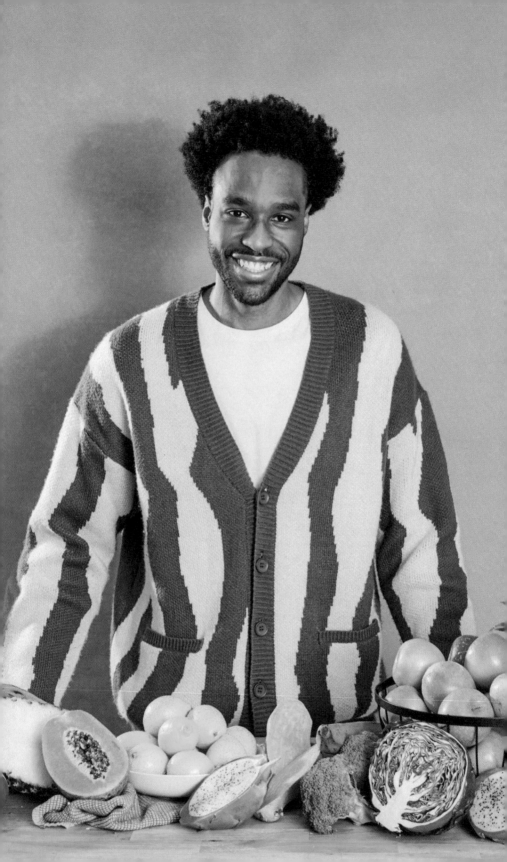

PHYSICAL WELLNESS: OPTIMIZING YOUR TEMPLE

Working on yourself internally is always paramount. The work has to start from within in order for any real change to take place. In addition to the internal transformation, it is key to home in on how you can facilitate that approach in the physical body and your immediate environment. The word of this section is *optimize* because that is the goal for the physical body and environment. I include environment because that can be just as influential if not more than any practice you want to take on. The space you inhabit is nothing more than an extension of both your physical and mental state and the aim of this section is to get you more clued into how you can optimize your physical self and space to yield best practices and results.

Everything is connected. How you treat your body can positively or negatively impact your mind and vice versa. We have a symbiotic relationship with the world around us and within us. The mind-body connection is often overlooked because they are viewed as two separate things and while they function independently, the link between them is what gives you more power, awareness, and strength in your day-to-day life to actualize more of what you want to create.

The word of this section is *optimize*, and the standard definition is "to make the best or most effective use of a situation, opportunity, or resource." This is the goal of operating in the physical or material world. Think about it—wouldn't you want to get the most pay out of your job for the least amount of effort? Or would you rather be swamped all the time and feel like you have to grind for everything you earn? This is not a trick question and it does not imply that you are lazy or do not care about your work and responsibilities. Things take effort, time, and energy, and we would be remiss to claim that putting more effort than necessary is what we would like to do, despite how glorified it is to be "hustling" or "making moves" all the time. Anyone can appreciate efficiency over the course of working on any endeavor. The goal is always to finish, actualize, accomplish, and achieve, not aimlessly working without a clear means to what you are doing to serve your interests. This is where optimization comes into play and where laziness can help you over the long haul.

An idea that comes to mind when discussing this is the term (originally coined by *The 4-Hour Workweek* author Tim Ferriss but adapted by Nike master trainer Joe Holder, who I learned it from) "strategic laziness." It is the idea that you only focus on what will advance you in whichever pursuit you take on. Being "lazy" in the sense of not opting for extra work just for the sake of it and synthesizing your practice to be the most efficient it can be. For example, high-level athletes train in a strategically lazy manner. They don't do anything outside what serves them in their specific sport; this is key to performance. For example, LeBron James needs to have a level of conditioning to sustain an eighty-two-game NBA season plus the postseason. The level of conditioning and miles run on the court amass to hundreds, if not thousands, over the course of a season. It is almost as if he's running marathons, but does that mean he needs to run an actual marathon to build that conditioning or train like an endurance runner? Absolutely not. Running and training for that marathon would only increase wear and tear on the body in addition to whatever other regimen was being taken on to prepare for his sport-specific performance. Athletes do only what is necessary to optimize their output and serve their goal because they know extra and wasted efforts can yield missed opportunities.

How do wasted or extra efforts yield missed opportunities, you might ask? Opportunities can be missed because there is not enough space for them to come through. If your head is always in the sand, plunging away at all this work and effort, you will never have the chance to look up and take in what might be presenting itself to you. For one, you will always be preoccupied, and two, your personal bandwidth will be drained so it will be hard to recognize something you might want to engage in further, even if it is more desirable.

It is important to keep the channels of creation as clear as possible so that when something you want presents itself, you can take full advantage and give it your best effort because you allocated your energy to afford you the ability to do so. There are many ways to accomplish a goal and many roads leading to the same destination, but oftentimes the scenic route may be the longest way to get there. It may seem appealing or look the best from the outside looking in and it could be nice to say you did it, but the priority is getting to the destination as soon as you can.

Even with this focus on the destination in sight, this does not take away from the importance of what it means to be present in the process overall. Yes, the aim is to get to the goal and we would want to optimize as many elements that we know we can to get us there as efficiently as possible, but the process is the practice. The goal is a split-second of an experience but the process is the day-in and day-out experience. It is what allows you to lean into that split-second goal feeling even more. It is the means to the end that is the goal or the vision. And it may even sound cliché always hearing "trust the process," and I would admit it is annoying to hear when you are in the thick of it, but it is all you can do.

Think about how often you have been faced with uncertainty and you did not know how something was going to come together. It was stressful and seemed like the most important thing at the time, yet here you are. You have made it on the other side and things came together for the best, didn't they? The moment either arranged itself better than you anticipated or maybe it didn't, but the actual moment was easier to face than imagined. Maybe you learned in hindsight that how it came together, even if it wasn't what you wanted originally, lends a lesson you carry with you now. Things usually unfold as they should and we cannot control everything. There is only so much you can do at a given point, and other people, circumstances, and elements must align to assist you in addition to your efforts, so this is where trusting the process comes into play.

This also goes back to keeping track of your personal highlight reel. The imagined scenario will almost always be more intense than the real moment. In the moment, instincts take over, what you have rehearsed takes precedence, or the truest and rawest form of you comes out and you don't think about when it is happening. Setting your intention for the process and following through on executing and optimizing it for the best results is how you see the effects of those efforts for the moments we face.

Mindful Movement

Working out, moving your body, exercising: whatever you want to call it, we can all agree it's objectively good for you, regardless of your relationship with it. Engaging in physical activity has many forms and benefits, but I am not necessarily here to tell you working out is good for you but rather to reframe what it means to have a movement practice and how it can amplify other areas of your lifestyle.

My relationship with working out was always through the lens of a high-achieving athlete. When I was playing basketball, every time I moved my body, it had to serve a purpose in regard to how I performed when it was game time. Whether it was a full-blown practice session with the team or a light stretch on a recovery day everything had to have a purpose, everything had to mean something and everything was thought to be the thing that made the difference between performing well or not. So, you could say the stakes were higher than usual. It wasn't until I came out of college basketball that I began to reexamine this thinking around movement.

As an athlete, you never have dominion over the relationship to what movement you identify with most. The focus is to perform and while in the midst of a season or preparation in the offseason, having the programming of your regimen outsourced frees your mind and allows you to focus only on doing the best you can. Having total dominion over your relationship with movement isn't always necessary in this context, and while it is useful at the time, it is rare that one would have the chance to foster that connection at all until leaving the sport. Coming out of this dynamic as an athlete to an everyday person can be jarring. If you always had someone to take care of preparing what you would do to serve your goals, it can leave you feeling lost regarding how you move your body outside of the context of a specific sport. Working out at the same rate and intensity isn't as sustainable for everyday life if you are not training for something specific and you have to discover what it means for you to maintain a movement practice if you even want to do that, given how much it has been structured until that point.

This is something I had to face upon choosing to step away from the game. I can say this looking back now but luckily, the injury I had forced me to rework how I trained and made me think deeper about what it meant to train for myself. From adopting more functional movement-focused workouts, to prioritizing strengthening the core, to developing more full-body connectivity, I was engrossed in an overhaul of what I knew it meant to be fit and strong. I learned in my recovery journey that muscle imbalances, having a weak core, and improper mechanics can lead to more injury, and it dawned on me that I had to start training for longevity and sustainability. Taking back some of that outsourced movement planning that a strength coach or trainer would have and being more intentional with how exercise affected me made a huge difference.

Even though I had been working out for most of my life, I never thought about how I wanted to feel or what I wanted to focus on as opposed to what I was told to do. Don't get me wrong—I needed the coaches and trainers as an athlete as I did not know everything about my body and needed some sort of guidance growing up but the injury offered me a seed of a perspective that I didn't know would carry into the rest of my movement journey, which is that having a mind-body connection is more important than any exercise you could do.

This touches on the idea of finding your why. Why do you want to work out? What do you feel it would do for you? What are your goals? How do you want to feel? Connecting to what you want to get out of the experience is the anchoring factor that allows a foundation to be built and practice to be established. This approach is the first step in creating a mind-body connection. The link that puts more intention into each form of movement you take on.

There are a lot of preconceived notions about exercising, most of which are intimidating and can sometimes scare people who may be on the fence about getting started or who have just started. A lot of what is shown about working out or gym culture is that everything has to be intense, everything you lift has to be heavy, and at the end of it you have to look a certain way, and if you don't do it this way, then you are not doing it right. It is framed as if this is the only way to do it. There is also the thought that every session has to be long and you have to be exhausted afterward and you have to be working out for hours to see results or to deem the session worthy. While this is an aspect of training that people take on, they do it because they want to, it is connected to their why. Yours may not look like this or it could be similar. Either way, knowing how you want to feel, above all, is the best place to start.

In starting or adapting a movement practice, you have to know there are options. Maybe a two-hour lifting session is not your bag, but, regardless of what you choose to take on, three main pillars of movement are paramount to success.

Longer Doesn't Mean Better

Get the idea out of your mind that every workout has to leave you drenched in sweat and barely able to walk afterward because that is not the only way to have an effective session. On top of that we all have stuff going on. Things take up space in our lives and sometimes we don't always feel we could allocate time to something physically challenging, being that everything else we're responsible for is just as challenging but in other areas like the mental or emotional sides. While that's all reasonable, we still need to get work in. We need to have an outlet for all that pent-up energy that comes from areas like work or home life or relationships. Ultimately it is time for you and only you.

Introducing the idea of *exercise snacks*. This is a concept birthed from a 2014 study that showed that three smaller sessions of exercise throughout the day (for around twelve minutes each) was more effective at lowering blood sugar and keeping it lower during the day than one longer thirty-minute session. So, don't stress if you don't have the time to have a longer dedicated session. You also don't have to do three sessions a day, but this goes to show that something is better than nothing. It also does not have to be complex. Sometimes this snack could mean light stretching and cardio, or you could set up a strength circuit and repeat a few movements for fifteen to twenty minutes. Aside from the physical benefits, you'll feel good that you took the time for yourself mentally, which makes it easier to keep up the habit.

Don't Skip the Routine, Build the Habit

Part of what will strengthen your practice will be building a habit of carving out time for yourself, working it into your routine and making it a priority. Each session will get easier to get into because you started the last one and, on those days, where you don't feel like doing it, having prioritized it before will make it easier to work through those feelings. Plus, you know it is a positive contribution to your everyday life.

I used *habit* and *routine* here, which for the most part I assumed were the same thing but they, in essence, are two separate things. One leads to the other. In a 2021 Harvard Business Review article by Kristi DePaul called "What Does It Really Take to Build a New Habit?" Nir Eyal, author of *Indistractable: How to Control Your Attention and Choose Your Life*, shared the difference:

> "A habit is a behavior done with little or no thought, while a routine involves a series of behaviors frequently, and intentionally, repeated. A behavior has to be a regularly performed routine before it can become a habit at all."

Most of us want to skip the routine phase, the part that is a little uncomfortable. Integrating a new behavior can be difficult. When we are hard-wired for so many other habits that keep us locked in a state of comfort or familiarity, it makes it hard to introduce something new that might uproot that comfort, even if it means what we were participating in before is something we don't want to continue. To get to that place where it doesn't feel like a chore every time you decide to move your body, you must go through the phase where it does. It has to mean more to you that you'll be honoring yourself and doing something to improve your quality of life over feeling that small discomfort at the start.

Produce Positive Stress

Keeping things concise and building habits are the more concrete parts of the process when it comes to elevating your physical well-being. One of the byproducts is you'll feel so much better. Think about a workout you had where you felt worse about yourself afterward. Outside of feeling sore or physically challenged (which doesn't always feel good), I'd be hard-pressed to think there were any times you felt like it was not worth it to take that step for yourself on an emotional or mental level. It's proven that exercise can boost neurochemicals like dopamine and serotonin that are associated with being in a good mood. You may not feel this as you're going through your workout session as the physical activity spikes a stress response. Think about it—if you're running a few miles, lifting heavy weights, or holding a yoga pose for a while, that's all stressful to the body. It expends energy to achieve a difficult task. Breaking down muscle tissue and raising your heart rate are conducive to stress. But we need that stress. It builds up the body's tolerance for that kind of experience and allows for a new threshold to be formed, making the next experience like that easier to handle.

Overall, stress is healthy but take note of two kinds of stress. *Distress* is associated with negative experiences like being overwhelmed or facing a difficult situation on any front—physical, mental, or emotional. This kind of stress sets in when the level of stress doesn't match the capacity you have to face it. *Eustress* is the other side of that coin, linked to positive experiences. "Positive stress?" you may ask. Yes, it exists, and you feel it more often than you think. Eustress is associated with spikes in the nervous system about something you may be excited about like a new project you're taking on, meeting a new romantic interest, or anticipating a vacation. Completing a challenging workout falls into this category. The chemicals it produces are feel-good ones like those other scenarios. Eustress is linked to being out of your comfort zone and conquering new challenges. This is the feeling you have after a workout and will positively link these occurrences in your mind, making them seem not so scary or intimidating.

I know for me, as long as I have been an active person, the workouts and doing the exercises never feel good. If anything, those are some of the last sensations I'd want to be feeling, but if one thing has kept me consistent with it, it's that eustress feeling. Aside from feeling good that the session is done, it feels amazing to know you're making progress. Feeling like I can run farther, jump higher, and lift more is a reminder that the stress is worth persevering through. It's real-time proof that the work is paying off. Unrelated to physical activity, this sensation is available through many mediums. Like finally getting past that writer's block, meeting a compatible romantic partner, or earning a promotion at work. All your efforts before then were the stressors you needed to persevere and see progress come to fruition. Again, it doesn't always feel good to go through it, it can be uncomfortable, painful, stressful, and everything in between, but the commitment to yourself makes it worth it along the way. So, transmute that distress into eustress!

You're Only as Good as Your Environment

You could do all this work on yourself, from managing your thought patterns to looking after your physical body and nourishing yourself with healthy foods, but your efforts could remain futile if your surroundings don't reflect what you are looking to achieve. Think about it—if you plant a rose in a desert, how would you expect it to grow? When it doesn't grow, would you say it's the rose's fault inherently? Was there something wrong with the seed or flower? Or was it the environment it was planted in that contributed to that result? The rose seed has everything within it needed to blossom into a beautiful flower, but its environment was not conducive to helping it actualize that form. The same goes for us and our blossoming.

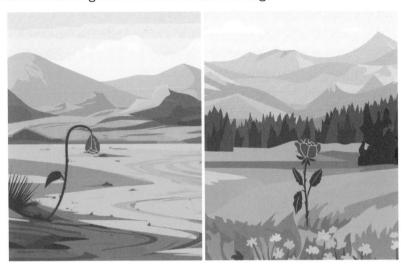

One of the greatest examples of how your environment affects your well-being is the idea of blue zones, a term coined by Dan Buettner, a National Geographic explorer. The concept grew from Gianni Pes and Michel Poulain, who were doing demographic work in Sardinia, Italy, where they found the highest concentration of male centenarians in the world. From their extended work in this field they drew blue circles around areas they found were hotspots for longevity, eventually calling them "blue zones."

Blue zones are great examples of this idea because these environments around the world are tangibly contributing to longer life and high-quality life. In these places a few common themes thread longevity together. They are more remote, far from the modernized world and its hustle, eliminating a big stress factor. The people rally around each other and have a true community. They support others as if they were family, yielding a great sense of belonging among the group. We need this as humans. Movement is ingrained into everyday activities like gardening, walking consistently, and group classes. The low-intensity movement done for hours each day keeps a level of fitness accessible into later years of life. They eat local, unprocessed, nutrient-dense foods native to their region. Often these diets consist of whole-food plant-based ingredients with minimal animal products, which is contrary to what we hear is most healthy for you. These environments make the healthy choice the easy one, the accessible one, and one that you don't have to think about because it is woven into the fabric of how you live. This is how you can set up your environment on a smaller scale to yield the results you want.

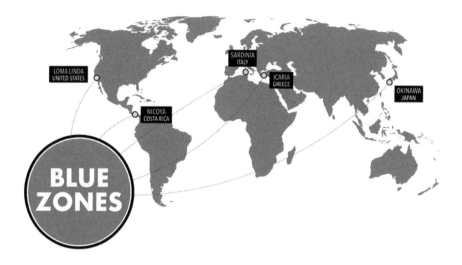

While all of our intentions, desires, and even actions may be aligned with a certain outcome, like getting a promotion at work, eating healthier, or staying consistent with a new routine, we can't do it all alone. We need help from outside sources. People have to come into your life, circumstances have to shift, and one way or another you will need to rely on something bigger than yourself to see the vision all the way through. One of these outside factors you can influence is your immediate environment.

Your home, workspace, car, or anywhere you inhabit space is an area you can set up so that it reflects what you want to achieve and enhances or streamlines your efforts to free your personal bandwidth around making decisions throughout the day. We all have a certain threshold for how much energy we put into making decisions in a day, from what to eat, what errands to run, where we have to go, how to get certain things done on time, the list goes on. These micro-decisions can be draining over the course of a day or week without proper optimization and preparation. Think about how less stressful your morning is when you lay out your clothes the night before as opposed to trying to pick a satisfactory outfit in the morning when you are in a rush and half asleep. Why not free up some of that space by optimizing your environment?

For example, let's say you have a goal to drink more water throughout the day. Without the proper optimization you might be stressed as to how much you need to drink, where you're getting the water from, how to make it cost-effective, etc. Having so much energy in these different places makes it more difficult to stick with the initial goal and attend to the important areas that need your direct attention. You would be going in blind to a new goal without having mapped out enough of how this can seamlessly integrate into your routine.

To properly set up your environment for success you'd need to know how much water you want to be drinking, always keep a reusable water bottle on you, make sure your home is stocked with water, maybe keep a glass by your bedside, even set up reminders on your phone for when to drink more. In this case, you don't have to actively think about where your water intake is coming from. Small changes to your surroundings make it easier to remember and always put you in a position to follow through on your goal with these little nudges from your environment. It would be so easy to falter on this path if, for instance, you didn't keep a water bottle on you, you ordered a soda every time you went out to eat, or there was no water in your living space. The goal is the same but one set of conditions makes it easier to execute than the other. This is what it means to know you're only as good as your environment.

When I think about this idea, I think about the nature-versus-nurture debate. But I feel there is no debate. It is not an *either/or* space; it is an *and* space. Both contribute greatly to one's path and it is the combination of the two that can yield different results. In this case, I'm speaking to more of the nurture side. We all inherit things (nature) we know don't serve us at times, also a lot of things that do. At a certain point, what we want out of life clashes with what we inherit, for better or worse. At this point, we have to tap more into the nurture side and create an environment, mindset, and vision for ourselves to form a new way of operating that ultimately shapes who we are. That's what taking accountability over the physical context you frame yourself in is all about.

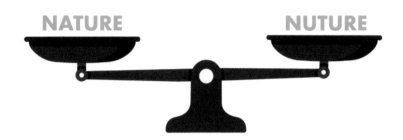

If you think about it, every sector of the society we live in now is set up this way, from government branches to school systems to production design. It is all designed to make efforts efficient. These are systems in place to alleviate sheer willpower and effort. Even with our access to information today. Could you even imagine going to the library, sifting through endless shelves, and dedicating hours to finding a book on a topic you'd want to research? Absolutely not. That amount of effort has been streamlined and optimized so we don't have to think about how to track down information anymore. Now it is just a few keystrokes away. Or with something as revolutionary as the assembly line. When Ford implemented the assembly line, production rates skyrocketed and reshaped the production industry as we know it. The reallocation of efforts and resources broke the process down into more manageable segments so less energy was spent trying to build a whole car at once. Rather, the assembly line focused on optimizing each step of the process, simplifying the workload, and specializing tasks so more could get done and be sustained over a longer period.

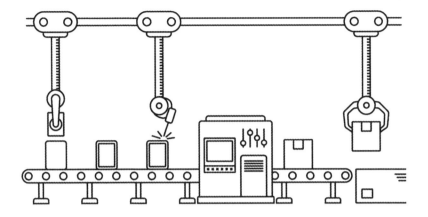

Treat your life like this assembly line and design the blueprint for your optimization. Examine what areas could use improvement and how you might set it up so you ultimately have to do less (strategic laziness). Look to design your life in a way that suits your vision at large but makes things easy on the ground level. Specialize tasks and delegate the workload to other tools you have available. You probably are already actively designing other areas of your life without knowing it. The simplest example might be setting an alarm for the morning. You're not concerned with having to wake yourself up at a certain time because you've outsourced that task to your alarm clock. Or you might meal prep so you don't have to think about what you'll be eating throughout the week with your busy schedule; this way you ensure you get a satisfactory meal every day. All these things play into tangibly making a change for the better. But again, the blade cuts both ways. If you, for instance, want to cut down on refined sugar but keep buying sugary cookies and cakes during your weekly grocery shop, it's harder for you to avoid eating them due to proximity since they are in your house and accessible. Proximity is power in the immediate environment and when you don't have it set up how you want, that proximity could be your greatest ally or greatest enemy.

When I think about this, I'm taken back to my basketball experience. My college coaches used to say, "At the end of the shot clock, you go to your bread and butter." For those that don't know, in basketball each team has a certain amount of time to take a shot each time they have

Section 2: Physical Wellness

possession of the ball. Each possession is measured by a shot clock, which varies in length depending on what level you play (high school, college, professional), anywhere from twenty-four seconds to thirty-five seconds. What my coaches meant by this is when the shot clock is dwindling and you have to take a shot, rarely will you perform a move or play that you have only practiced a few times. It is more likely that you will revert to something you are more familiar with, something you've done a million times and is second nature. At this time, all thinking goes out the window and you are operating on muscle memory and instincts. The same goes for our personal decision threshold. When we are tapped out and need to decide from this space (when the shot clock is winding down), the first, most familiar, and most available option will likely be the one we choose because it is convenient. The element of life design comes into play when we can make those most familiar and available options the ones we know benefit us the most in relation to how we want to live.

One of the biggest adjustments I made in my life around this area was when I decided to go plant-based and stay consistent with it. I loved the way I felt and I knew I wanted to continue so I had to think of how I could best set myself up for success when I was in unfamiliar territory. This meant I had to stock up on foods in my living space that supported my goal of staying plant-based. At the time, this living space was my college dorm. Fresh fruits and veggies weren't widely available on campus outside of school hours but with my schedule and demand on my body as an athlete, my teammates and I would need more access to food after hours. On top of that, freshly made food was hard to come by after a certain time. For me this meant loading up on all the fresh produce and hearty plant-forward meals I could during the school day from the dining hall. I carried anywhere from three to five plastic Tupperware containers in my backpack daily to store second and third helpings of whatever I was eating to bring it back to my dorm for later on. I knew if I didn't take this step, it would be hard for me to stay as consistent as I would like and could lead to me reaching for the most convenient options like junk and fast food just to stay satiated in the later hours of the day or not eating enough altogether.

This tactic stays with me to this day. Aside from the many to-go containers on my person, anywhere I go that takes me out of my routine or normal eating environment is grounds for preparation. If I'm traveling I'll always load up on fresh fruits and hydrating juices from local markets to ensure I can sustain energy levels and continue to consume healthy foods on the go. I look at menus for restaurants in the area and pin down places I know I can go that fit how I want to eat, even if it means I'm diverting from my group of friends or family for a meal or two.

This is not the case every time, but taking accountability for my environment, loading up on info and a base level of goods needed to keep my decision threshold free allows me to have my "bread and butter" already in place if the shot clock gets low, therefore keeping me always aligned with my goals. "That sounds like a lot of work," you might be saying. And yes, at first, it is. Learning how to take care of yourself in the way you want takes work. Building trust and reliance on your instincts, motivations, and intentions is a full-time job and there is no getting around it, but the work you put into this job pays you back in peace of mind, aligned actions, and feeling good.

If you want a simpler task, here is a pro tip: Take advantage of your lock and home screens on your devices. This is *extremely* underrated. We look at these things countless times throughout the day, so why not have the first thing you see be calming, grounding, affirming, or motivating? I started changing my wallpaper to short affirmations when initially taking an audit of my physical environment, either that or calming images like "I am," "Live at the edge of your capabilities," "Be the space," "cosmic alignment," and more. It varied based on the point of emphasis in my journey at that time. Constantly being reminded every time I looked at my phone offered more peace than I anticipated. Right now, I don't have one on my wallpaper but I have a reminder set to alert me every day: "Embody what you want to experience. You have it already. You are a powerful creator." This is my focus and it helps to have that reminder daily. Aside from that, our devices are probably our biggest sources of stimulation. So, before you doom scroll for hours or approach the many notifications you get in a day, use the wallpaper to offer you some sort of peace beforehand. I promise this helps more than you think.

During the hustle and bustle of daily life it becomes harder to consciously make these decisions about everything. We all have a threshold and when we meet that threshold, things go into autopilot, meaning we do the bare minimum to get by until our vital energy can replenish. The goal of optimizing your environment is to positively automate those autopilot decisions. Society would have us believe that everything must be hard, as exerting so much effort to get something done is glorified these days. While some effort does have to be put in, it may not be as much as you think. Things shake out how they would anyway, regardless of our efforts. Sometimes we end up running in place, thinking we have a grasp on the outcome when there are so many other factors at play.

Something that shifted my perspective on this is a section from spiritual thought leader and bestselling author Deepak Chopra's book, *The Seven Spiritual Laws of Success.* The fourth chapter, titled "The Law of Least Effort," concisely sums up what it means to be able to do less and still get what you want and maybe more.

"If we observe nature at work we see that the least effort is expended. Grass doesn't try to grow; it just grows. Fish don't try to swim; they just swim. This is their intrinsic nature. It is the nature of the sun to shine. And it is human nature to make our dreams manifest into physical form—easily and effortlessly."

This is key to optimizing your environment. By understanding some things will be what they will be and there is no need to try and convince anyone or take control all the time. It becomes grounding and humbling to know we don't have control over everything we'd like to. It is a huge check to our ego that demands we impose our will over a given circumstance. There is great power in taking solace over knowing you did all you could do and letting the rest reveal itself. "Least effort is expended when our actions are motivated by love, because nature is held together by the energy of love," Chopra states. In other words, all the action needed will be inspired action. You will simply feel the need to take a certain step at a certain time and it will be clear where to direct your energy, which is exactly where you want to be. When operating from a space of openness and being tuned in to your guidance system, you will always feel good about the progress you're making.

To set yourself up for success in your immediate environments you need structure. Here are some of the best tips I've implemented when making my surroundings reflect my goals:

Build Your Assembly Line

Setting up your environment for optimization will require you to perform an audit on what can use improvement in your current surroundings. In thinking about the assembly line analogy, what tasks can you delegate to other tools (like the alarm clock)? What do you know you need to do but need reminders to stay on track? How can you make what you want to have access to when your decision threshold is being met ready and accessible so you don't have to think about it?

Little by little you will begin to find small hacks and tricks that add up to a well-oiled machine that is your assembly line. The things you can offload from your conscious efforts make a huge difference in the long haul when you have a bigger, more time-consuming task in front of you. Delegating tasks when you can allows you to free up mental and physical space, making you more available to prioritize what you need. With this method you become less concerned with building a whole car in one go but rather executing each task with the most efficiency and placing the focus there. The result is a fully functional vehicle.

Proximity Is Power (Bread and Butter)

Proximity is power and I think this is an underrated element of making any lifestyle change. Like the example of refined sugar, what is closest, most available, and familiar will be the default option in a crunch. When the decision threshold has been crossed, your vital energy drained, and you want to turn off your brain, you want to know you're safe to make mindless decisions and not feel like your goals are at risk. The real reward is making these decisions and having them serve you just as much as if you were consciously seeking out the healthiest dish or lowest-effort task.

Begin to look around your environment, living space, car, and workplace. What is most available? What is most familiar? Do these things serve your interests? If so, then you can afford to turn your brain off at times and know what you reach for in any context is safe. If not, you might have to dedicate more energy than you want to at a given time to ensure you are aligned with your intentions or run the risk of compromising out of convenience.

Stop Trying

Yes, you read that correctly. Stop trying so hard. We can only control so much in the external world. The real key is identifying what you can control. We can never control another person's reaction to something, how what we say is interpreted, what the traffic will be like, or when the next goal of yours will arrive. What we can do is look at what is within our control, like how we choose to react and interpret, manage our internal state, as well as look at our immediate environment to see what we can change so it reflects who and what we know ourselves to be.

Every change to the physical environment also doesn't have to be a hack to complete a task. Sometimes it could be a small affirmation written on a notepad at your desk or a calming image on your phone lock screen that grounds you every time you go to open it: anything that gets you to loosen your grip on the day. Once we manage what we can, it helps to release and let the rest take shape.

If you place your order how you like at a restaurant, do you then feel the need to go back into the kitchen and prepare it yourself? No. You trust the staff will deliver your order as you requested. That's what taking control of what you can feels like, knowing you did what you could and allowing the rest to be shown to you. Apply the Law of Least Effort and be like nature. Let it unfold and stay aligned with your intuition:

"Attention to the whims of the ego consumes the greatest amount of energy. But when our internal reference point is our spirit, our actions are motivated by love, and there is no waste of energy."

—Deepak Chopra, *The Seven Spiritual Laws of Success*

The Productivity of Presence

When we set out on a path to get something done, it is an active pursuit. Our efforts take time and energy, both of which we can't get back once expended. There is a lot of hype around productivity these days. It is all about how much you can get done in the quickest amount of time. The more you get done the more valuable you seem. While it is important to get as much done as you can that aligns with your goal, an area that gets overlooked is the quality of engagement we have with our everyday tasks as opposed to the quantity.

Taking more time to re-center and ground within each task throughout your day can yield dividends in the areas of mental, emotional, and physical well-being. Mentally, your brain can be more at ease and focus on what you want, stripping away all the chatter and extra things to think about that pull your attention in a million different directions. The emotional and physical I view as more interconnected. Our emotional state has a direct effect on what our body experiences. The body itself is a blank slate; it is literal. It autonomously does what it needs to function optimally but aside from that it responds to what we feed it, which can enhance or diminish the feedback you get from it.

If you take a second now to recall a moment when you felt happy— maybe it was a gathering with loved ones, receiving a nice gift, or eating your favorite food. Think about that time, take yourself back; how did it feel? When you did that just now, your recalling of emotions from a happy time had a physical ripple effect. You might have felt butterflies in your stomach or your muscles released tension for a moment, your breathing slowed down, and maybe a slight smile grew on your face. Your body responded to the input you gave it and that was a feel-good experience. You knew mentally and logically that it was just a memory, but the body doesn't know the difference. All it received was information to produce the same chemicals and sensations as if it were happening in real-time. This is one of the many ways presence can change your outer-world experience.

When you are in pursuit of your goals in the day-to-day grind, call upon your ability to root yourself in whatever you are doing, even if it is tedious (I'd say even more so in those times). It can be easy to check out when things are not where or what we think they should be; it seems to be easier if we disconnect until it is all over, but remember what was mentioned about habits? If you regularly implement the behavior of checking out, it becomes part of your routine. The active implementation over time builds an association and soon becomes an unconscious habit because you are resistant to the circumstance. This makes it harder to be where you are and truly sink into the quality of your experience.

Slow living comes to mind when accounting for more presence in everyday life. It is the idea that decelerating the pace at which we take on our daily tasks can bring about more peace and build a better relationship to the process of productivity. Slow living is not as much of a process as it is an approach, a life philosophy. It affords you the opportunity to frame the practice of presence within a set idea, which might make it easier to integrate into your daily life.

From a conventional lens, productivity and presence don't seem like they would align. They seem like two ends of the spectrum based on common associations. Productivity, on one end, is traditionally seen as something that lends itself to more intensity, hustle, and effort while presence is more associated with stopping, slowing down, and inaction. Having one does not mean you cannot have the other. Getting anything done will require that you expend energy and focus on the tangible means to actualize that goal. At times this may look like the conventional productivity view. This is also not a bad thing, as it is the inherent nature of the process. The key is finding ways to bring presence into the fold while the hustle is happening in real-time. This could be as small as stopping whatever you are doing and taking one deep breath if things get overwhelming, then continuing. Another way is taking in all your senses—how do objects feel in your hands? What do you hear or smell? This is one of the quickest ways to root into the now. It can also be as intentional as setting aside time in your day for mindful reflection, self-regulation, meditation, and realignment as a longer, more substantial session may work better for you.

A combination of both helped me regulate the hustle. Once I started to become aware of how much effort I was putting out was draining and overwhelming me (in the midst of handling the responsibilities of being a student-athlete, along with recovering from my injury) altering how I approached the day-to-day grind helped shift my health on all levels. I started using mundane tasks as an entry point to peace. Taking in all the sights and sounds on my walks to class and the gym, to sitting and eating my meals with no external stimulation like my phone to distract me. I made the intention to take in the company I had with me or if I was by myself, just being comfortable in that.

I even brought this into my workouts, recovery routine, and physical activity. Ultimately, this helped me establish a way better relationship with my body because of how much I was tuned in to how everything felt, the good and the bad. Both are necessary and exposure to both expands your capacity to identify which is which and how much you can withstand. A lot of the time, when doing physical activity, it is easy to go into autopilot. Because you know you have a target rep count or time frame to perform the movement, that's all you focus on is getting to that as fast as possible. This is a great analogy for life challenges. You know where you want to go, and you would like to get there as quickly and easily as possible. But the process of getting there is challenging and uncomfortable, much like doing those exercises. The exercises are not meant to be comfortable; they are meant to build strength, resilience, and stamina. You cannot build these new areas of growth without breaking down the old ones first.

As my physical activity rate decreased dramatically since having the surgery, plus having to rebuild strength and mobility in my ankle, I had to start from square one with my body. Initially, I found this stressful because every way I knew how to train was thrown out the window. I was tasked with having to find a new way to build my body back up and with some help from the internet, the training staff at school, and my health mentor, I could integrate a new level of mindfulness into my productivity around exercise and recovery.

It was reframing what it meant to be strong. The idea most of us have when we think about strength is about lifting the most weight; while that is a dimension of strength, there are so many other ways to be strong. If you see a yoga teacher hold a handstand or a gymnast stick a dismount, that's all strength! I started to approach my regimen like one of those athletes as opposed to a traditional basketball player. When we have these target reps we aim for when exercising, we want to just get it over with and do it as fast as we can, but I have found when you slow down the movement and tune in to that uncomfortable feeling that is a pushup or a squat, then your mind and body learn how to better navigate that sensation, ultimately building more strength. Slow training is beneficial because of *time under tension*.

This places your body under tension for longer, making your muscles work harder to support you through movement. Overall, you perform fewer reps with this method but increase the working time you would have with a conventional training method. This is where mindfulness comes in. To perform, for example, a squat for five seconds down and five seconds up forces you to stay present with the movement and stay with the weight all the way through because there is no quick escape like performing the same move but faster to get it done. It is challenging, feeling the tension in your muscles as you go down slowly and back up and having to consciously engage different parts of your lower body establishes a mind-body connection that ultimately builds confidence in your ability to perform because you know to respond to the discomfort at each stage. Focusing on functional, intentional movements like this that translate to real-world activity made me a better-performing athlete and a better-performing human. Building a relationship with movement through incorporating intention is a huge part of my ability to make a full recovery at the time. Feeling less of the aches and pains when walking up a flight of stairs or sitting down for too long all melted away once these practices were implemented on a regular basis. The integration of mindfulness in this arena catapulted me to a new level of productivity.

Another area that gets overlooked in the culture of productivity is sleep or rest. Sleep is a basic human need; everyone knows this, yet at times it is the most taken for granted. "Sleep is for the weak" or "I'll sleep when I'm dead" are a few expressions that get tossed around in productivity culture that frame taking rest as a sign of weakness. In reality, without proper rest, your likelihood of embodying weakness is much higher. I get it—there are a lot of things to do and only so much time in the day. Sometimes the tasks at hand might spill over into the time you have allotted to rest. Occasionally, this won't hurt but if it becomes a habit to compromise your time to rest in the name of getting more done, then you might not get as much done as you'd like.

A 2010 study found that sleep disturbances significantly impacted worker productivity and ultimately cost employers almost $2,000 a day per employee for the lack of output based on unhealthy sleep patterns.[1] The lack of quality sleep spills over into other areas like mood regulation, immune system strength, memory, and cognition issues. Sleep is not just something we have to do each night because we are tired. It is the process necessary to carry out so many functions we are not even aware of. They require so much energy we can't even be awake for them to take effect. Just think, if you go to the gym or workout, you're not getting stronger in the workout itself. The workout breaks down the body, tearing muscle fibers and pushing to the limit of your conditioning. You don't get the benefits of the workout until after you have rested and recovered properly. The muscles repair themselves to withstand more resistance, making you stronger, and this all happens through resting.

In this case, if you're an active person but don't get adequate sleep, it would be hard for you to make the gains you are looking for. Loss of sleep promotes fat storage and decreased muscle growth. The body assumes due to lack of proper sleep that it is in a survival state, storing fat for energy reserves and prioritizing that over building muscles to exert more energy. So maybe the most important key to your goals is not even workout-related; it is based on how many hours you are clocking a night on a consistent basis. Why do you think babies sleep so much? They are developing so much physical matter within the first few years of life to allow them to function as full-grown humans that they need to be at rest most of the time. As an adult, you may not be developing as much as an infant but your amount of rest carries the same weight.

We develop so much through sleep based on our circadian rhythm, which is the internal body clock all living organisms have. Based on this rhythm, our body knows when to sleep, when to eat, when it can exert the most energy, and so on. This rhythm supports our every function in the body and it needs consistency to function optimally, therefore keeping us as sharp as we can be. This is why we get hungry around the same time every day, get sleepy around the same time, or have

1   Rosekind, Mark R., et al. "The Cost of Poor Sleep: Workplace Productivity Loss and Associated Costs." *Journal of Occupational and Environmental Medicine*, vol. 52, no. 1, 2010, pp. 91–98. JSTOR, http://www.jstor.org/stable/44998613. Accessed 5 Apr. 2024.

energy at certain parts of the day, to essentially make it easier for the body to know when it will receive these things, making it predictable so that it can stay efficient with its processes. If it was not made as predictable, we would always be out of sorts and not feel regulated on a consistent basis.

While our bodies take over the duties necessary that are aligned with this rhythm, it is still a malleable thing. We have the power over this rhythm in that we can establish a new one at any time. If you take a flight from Los Angeles to New York City, you most likely will get sleepier much later in the day once you've landed on the East Coast than you would on the West Coast because you're used to a certain rhythm and your body has to adjust. This is where you have an opportunity to manually adjust the circadian rhythm. The biggest and most useful tools to use when adjusting are all the major pillars of the circadian rhythm: sleeping, eating, and activity.

Our primary reference point for our bodies' rhythm is the sun. If the sun is out, you know you have to be up and active; when night falls, you know it is time to wind down and rest. It is an innate rhythm built within us and we can use it to our advantage when recalibrating. Use sun exposure to jumpstart your circadian rhythm. Even if you are not changing time zones or traveling, getting ten to fifteen minutes of sun exposure in the morning upon waking cues all the systems within to know it is time to be awake, thus starting the internal timer as to when it will be time to sleep. This all lends itself to better quality sleep at the end of the night because your body is cued accordingly. If you are traveling or adjusting to a new time zone, use the most accessible tool, the sun, to aid in your transition by following your routine as if it were the time of day wherever you came from.

Secondly, maintaining your eating schedule is key to circadian rhythm. We all typically have the same times we eat in a day; our body needs ample time to ingest and digest what we take in and that's why we eat when we do. Staying true to those natural cues further plays into your internal clock and lets your body know it is safe. This ultimately contributes to better sleep at the end of the day. Digestion does take a long time and requires a lot of energy, so a pro tip: try not to eat a big meal within two hours of going to bed. It might not always be possible but that is okay. If you exercise this practice the majority of the time, that's what matters. The energy required to process the food you took in can take away from energy needed for getting into deep REM sleep, making you less sharp upon rising.

Movement is another pillar you can use to regulate your rhythm. Incorporating a workout at a time when your circadian rhythm might be out of order is a great way to tell your body that you have expended a high amount of energy, making it easier for it to start winding down later after exerting itself. The endorphin and dopamine hit you get from a good sweat session is also a way to temporarily spike your energy level and wake yourself up, should you need it. As mentioned before, it doesn't have to be long. Something as quick as a ten- or fifteen-minute active stretching session to a twenty-five-minute strength or conditioning circuit will do the trick.

When you start coming down from the day, let yourself come down. Eliminate stimuli later in the night, like excess noise and light, to allow the brain more space to produce the neurochemicals needed to put you to bed. The screens, devices, lights, and background noise all give the brain a job and that job is to process all that input so you can perceive it, which is what it is designed for. Doing this into the hours right before bed could, in a way, trick your brain into thinking you still need to be awake and active. It may make the brain delay producing the melatonin you need to start falling asleep. If you think about a casino and how it is designed to keep people awake and alert, it is no accident people can be in there for hours on end. The lights are bright and colorful, hitting all the sensory input for your eyes to be engaged, the sounds are high-pitched and ever-present, making a quiet moment hard to come by. Not to mention the stimulation from whatever game a person might be playing. Occupying the brain with all these arousing elements makes it hard to focus on any one thing so it has been on and vigilant, keeping you awake in the process. So at the end of the night, dim the lights, turn the volume down, put away the screens, and give your brain less to process. This makes it easier to get the rest you need.

There is also something to be said about building these habits to lighten the load, should you go off track. Think about if you were learning to play the piano and you practiced every day for weeks on end. The consistency of the practice would result in gaining more skill and higher levels of performance. If you were to take a few days off, you wouldn't lose all your skill in those few days. The practice you have built keeps you at a set point to start from which you can pick right back up. The same goes for keeping our body and circadian rhythm in check. These core areas around the circadian rhythm can all cultivate better, more consistent sleep if practiced regularly. If we get more high-quality sleep on a regular basis, our productivity for life goes up, making it easier to show up how we want to. Most times, the approach to fixing sleep habits or any other ailment is to address the symptoms and not the root causes. The melatonin supplements or trying to force yourself to sleep only go so far. Making these adjustments in small increments in different areas of your life over time adds up to the dosage you need to address the overarching symptoms. A mindful approach like this is more sustainable and accessible than any prescription you could get.

There is a symbiotic relationship we have with nature as humans that is in the fabric of our everyday routine. Using the sun to cue the start of your day may seem rudimentary but there is an ancient wisdom ingrained in the use of such modalities to complement our modern world. Think about how much more tired or drowsy you feel if it is cloudy all day . The presence of the sun has a direct link to our physiological being. Everything on this planet is alive and working within a cycle of life we had nothing to do with and couldn't even if we wanted to. The cycle takes place among every living organism on the planet. If, for example, you take a tomato that gets planted from a small seed, it grows in living soil that provides it with nutrients to sprout, which eventually turns it into a full plant that bears many fruits. They get harvested and end up on our dinner table in whatever form we prepare. The nutrients that one seed absorbs in the ground transfer to us when we eat it. The waste from the plant goes right into compost, which fertilizes more soil to repeat the process. The air we breathe is generated by plants all around us and what we breathe out allows them to breathe and thrive, making for an invaluable exchange that keeps us and them alive.

Touching our bare feet to grass in a field or sand at the beach provides a link to the earth's reservoir of electromagnetic energy, which balances our negative and positive ion distribution and grounds us. Immersing yourself in nature for at least two hours a week has been shown to yield better health reports than those who didn't.[2] There is an interconnectedness between us and our natural environment that is directly tied to our health and well-being. Aside from the physical or mental benefits, taking time to soak these in and use them to our advantage puts us in a position to connect deeper with ourselves and introduce more mindfulness. Nature goes at its own pace and everything gets done on time. We could use that as a reminder to know our unfolding is in divine timing. Connecting to what is so deeply active in our life force is grounding and liberating. To know we are part of the same energy that are the giant redwoods or the myriad of species on the planet can be humbling. Using these small points of access, these small moments of mindfulness can give us what we need to be productive in the way we see fit.

Though a practice like this may seem super regimented at first, it allows more freedom than you might think despite the discipline and intention needed up front to get started. A few desserts here, a couple of days of rest there, will not nullify your progress. In fact, taking on such mindful habits affords you more freedom in these ways. You have a foundation built on knowing how to manage how you want to feel daily. Putting it into action productively, you now know exactly how much wiggle room you have to veer off the routine and not feel the setbacks as intensely or at all. That relationship you build with yourself through a mindful approach and showing up for yourself consistently yields the productivity you desire.

---

2   White, M.P., Alcock, I., Grellier, J. *et al.* Spending at least 120 minutes a week in nature is associated with good health and wellbeing. *Sci Rep* **9**, 7730 (2019). https://doi.org/10.1038/s41598-019-44097-3.

Use Anything to Access Presence

When I say "use anything to access presence," I mean *anything*. Find peace in the mundane and ordinary—pouring a glass of water, taking your daily commute, talking to a friend, listening to your favorite song. Anything can be a point of access to grounding into a mindful lifestyle. You don't have to force this or make everything a spiritual moment, but when you feel like you're on autopilot and become aware of it, using the small things around you to root back into the now will afford you the wherewithal to make more conscious decisions daily. Operating from this space gives you more access to make decisions from the highest level of consciousness, making you more productive along the way.

Sleep Is for the Strong

You wouldn't use your phone all day without charging it overnight or drive your car when the tank is on low, so you should be no different. Sleep keeps us sharp and fresh. Prioritize getting the amount and quality you need to be at your best. Take account of where your circadian rhythm is and if it needs adjusting. Take small daily habits and see how you could maximize them for optimal rest, from strategic sun exposure to what time you eat, to enacting a true wind-down routine before bed. All of these become the rhythm your body follows because this is what you told it was the preferred mode of operation. This circadian rhythm sets the tone for your day so make sure it is the tone you want.

Be with Nature

There is a wealth of innate intelligence within nature. Although modern society has wedged a divide between our connection to this, we are a part of this intelligence. We can actively participate in coherence with it so we can enhance what we would like to accomplish in our lives. Take some time to intentionally connect—sit in a park, walk barefoot, stargaze, and do something to ground you in the abundance we have at our disposal.

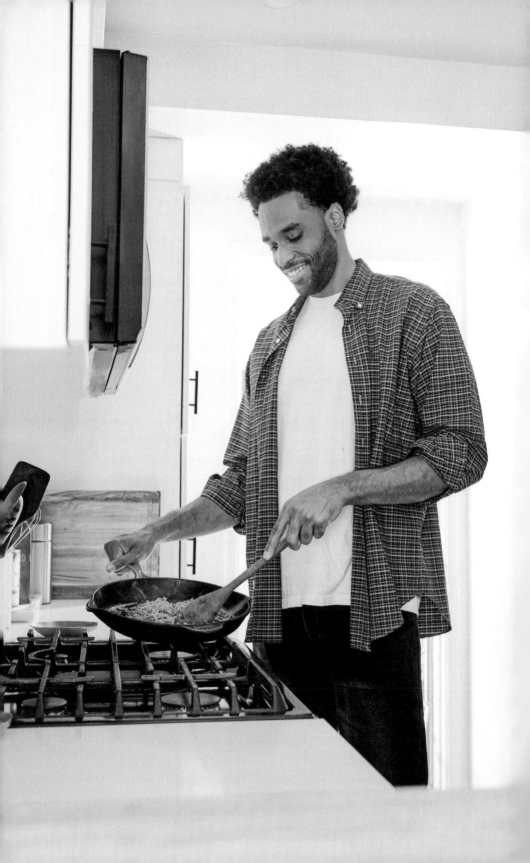

Section 3

NUTRITIONAL WELLNESS:

GAINING POWER TO PERFORM

All the work you do on yourself has to be fueled correctly. There is no secret that food supplies us with energy for our everyday life. At its core, food is information for our bodies. Based on what we consume, different responses are carried out. For example, if you eat a piece of bread mainly comprised of carbohydrates, the process needed for digesting and absorbing is different from what's needed to digest and absorb a bowl of chickpeas, which are mainly protein. Based on what you put in your body, you are essentially telling it what function to perform, what system to activate, and what action to carry out at any given time. In addition to the information you are inputting, there is an output at play that serves as feedback from that information we take in. Paying attention to the way you feel in response to what you are eating is the easiest way to gauge what might work best for you. We use certain foods and drinks like coffee, pressed juice, oatmeal, or a salad at different points to give us the energy response we are looking for during the day. The feedback we get from these things is what determines the quality of our day in most cases and while some may just think "food is food," tapping in to how this information you eat informs your life can be another growth point on your path to your highest self.

When I initially started paying attention to what I was eating and how it affected me was on the road to recovery from my injury in college. My health mentor, who was an NBA trainer at the time and plant-based, told me to try it out to see how I felt. It was more of an experiment than anything. All I knew was I was trying to get back to 100 percent to play again and would have done just about anything to get there. What started as a few days grew into weeks and then months. I started to feel lighter after meals and felt like I was gaining energy as opposed to feeling like I had to sit down for hours following a meal. Weight that I didn't know I was trying to lose fell off in the best way. It felt as if my body was optimizing itself right before my eyes. Aside from recovering quicker, having less inflammation, and physically healing, the biggest surprise from making the switch was how clear I felt mentally. I felt clearer than ever, sharp, and present and I had a deep understanding that this newfound power came from my lifestyle choices. If you've ever seen the movie *Limitless* starring Bradley Cooper in which he takes pills that unlock 100 percent of his brain capacity, it felt like that. It might sound outlandish but that is the best way to describe it.

Taking the onus upon yourself to make these kinds of decisions, especially with food, can have you feeling limitless. While I am plant-based, in no way does this mean going plant-based is the only way to be healthy. Everyone's body is different and responds to things differently than others. The most I could do is encourage you to take these steps below and find your balance regarding what it means for you to eat well (and try some of the recipes out while you're at it).

Feel-Good Food

Start paying attention to how food makes you feel physically after consumption, not just how good it makes you feel emotionally because of taste, convenience, etc. Understanding the feedback loop from the quality of food being consumed to the energy response you get from it and how that translates into the rest of your day is key to unlocking higher levels of understanding within yourself because you begin to learn your body and give it what it needs. This gives you a cheat code to get to a place where you can feel like Bradley Cooper in *Limitless*. Knowing what foods give you the best bodily response and compounding those choices each day make for a better you over time.

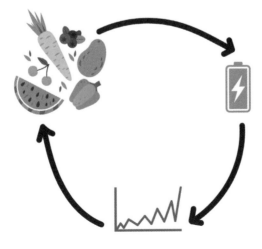

Whole Food Harmony

Regardless of your dietary preferences, there is no argument against eating foods with minimal to no processing and having them in their whole form. If you made no other changes besides removing the ultra-processed foods from your diet like refined sugar–filled sweets, fast food, and factory-farmed meat and replacing them with whole, organic, less processed options, you would see a significant change in that feedback loop. Aside from that, whole foods are more nutrient-dense. This might mean that you would be eating less naturally because your body is getting what it needs to feel satiated over time. Before there were ever vitamins, fitness fads, or trendy diets, there were whole foods—products of nature that give us everything we need to not only survive but thrive. Now we have more access than ever to these foods and luckily being healthy is in trend. So why not hop on the wave and get a few extra nutritionally sound ingredients from your local market?

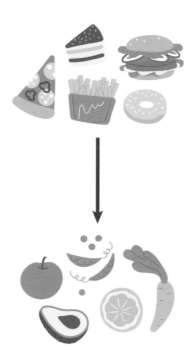

If You Can't Read It, Don't Eat It (Do Your Best)

If you do a little research you will find many options available for food products that have the same level of indulgence and satisfaction made with whole, clean ingredients as their processed counterparts. It is no secret at this point how the additives and chemicals in some of these foods negatively impact human health yet we still participate. Maybe it is because of comfort and familiarity or maybe it is because we don't know of other options or may not have access to them. No matter the case, if you are looking to make a shift to higher-quality foods, a general rule I'd recommend is, if you can't read it, don't eat it. This means to always read the ingredients on packaged foods to ensure you are getting the highest quality option. Things to look out for would be additives and ingredients that sound like they came out of a lab (because they probably did). Look out for gums, modified starches, and anything with a number next to it. If a food contains any or all of these, it might not be best to consume it on a regular basis, if at all. Stick to products with ingredients you can easily recognize, and the shorter the ingredients list, the better.

While this rule is straightforward, it is not 100 percent literal. Give yourself some grace when starting to shift your lifestyle and know you won't get it all figured out immediately, especially around diet. Too many people dive headfirst into the deep end without even learning to swim first, thinking that is the only way to make progress. Make the best choice you can from the point of understanding you have now, and the rest will unfold. If you are committed to a higher level of health, all the right elements will find you.

Quick Cravings

We all have busy lives. Whether you enjoy preparing meals for yourself or not, time is not always on our side regarding making something nourishing while we are pressed for time. All of these recipes come together in twenty minutes or less, so they're perfect for when you are in a pinch and are easy to prepare ahead of time to save yourself some energy in the future.

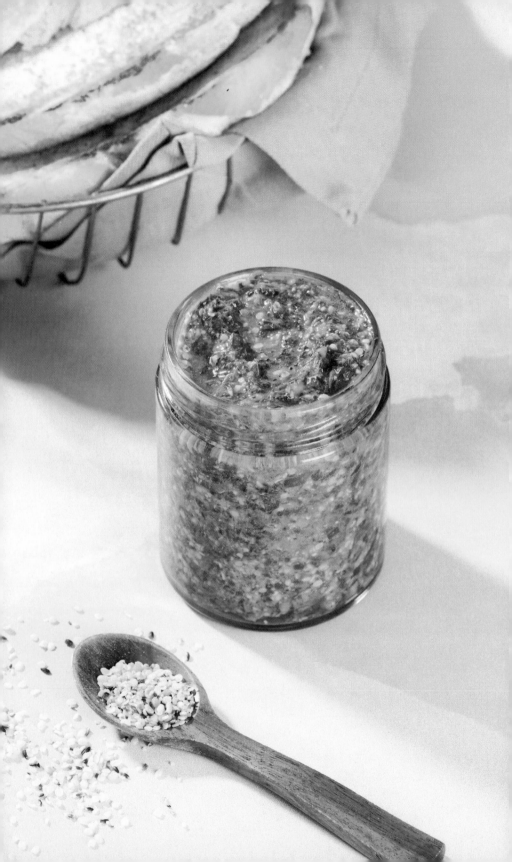

HEMP SEED PESTO

Ingredients

4 packed cups (200 g) fresh basil leaves

⅔ cups (80 g) nutritional yeast

juice of one lemon (approximately 45 g)

4 tablespoons (40 g) hemp seeds

3 garlic cloves

salt and pepper to taste

⅓ cup (79 mL) olive or avocado oil

This quick and easy pesto is a game changer. It was one of the first things I learned to make vegan and is a staple of mine to this day, I have a feeling it might be one of yours soon as well. It can go on pasta and salads, in stir-fries, and so much more. It's not traditional by any means but it's not supposed to be. It's a quick way to concentrate flavor and keeps in the fridge or freezer for a good while to enjoy.

Instructions

Add everything aside from the oil into a food processor. Process until combined.

Remove the lid and scrape down the sides with a spatula.

Place the lid back on and, with the food processor running, drizzle in the olive oil. Start with ¼ cup and add more if needed. Scrape down the sides a few times and process again until smooth.

Transfer to a glass container and store in the fridge for up 5 days or the freezer for up to 6 months.

NOT ANOTHER BLACK BEAN BURGER

Ingredients

1 cup (195 g) black or brown rice

½ onion (approximately 70 g)

4-5 mushrooms (approximately 80 g)

1 can (425 g) of black beans (drained and rinsed)

½ cup (48 g) gluten-free oats

1 tsp (6 g) salt

1 tsp (2 g) pepper

1 tsp (2 g) smoked paprika

1 tsp (3 g) garlic powder

1 tsp (3 g) onion powder

1 tsp (1 g) dried thyme

¼ cup (60 g) ketchup

You may think black bean burgers are basic or boring. But we all need those dishes that are consistent and this is that. When the right elements are enhanced, like flavor and texture, a black bean burger can be one of the most satisfying things to have. This is also a great base method for any legume-based burger you'd want to create. Swap out the legume itself or throw in different seasonings and you have a unique twist on a classic method.

Instructions

Start by cooking your rice to package instructions and set aside to cool (you can use day-old rice as well). Sauté your half onion with the mushrooms (roughly chopped) until onions are translucent and mushrooms have released all moisture. Mash black beans in a large bowl with a fork until the mixture resembles mashed potatoes with a few beans still intact. Blend ½ cup of oats and your spices in a food processor until granular and spices are incorporated. Mix mashed beans, sautéed vegetables, and cooked rice in a mixing bowl along with blended spice flour. Add ketchup to mixture. Mix until all combined and mixture forms a patty. Pan fry until crispy and cooked through. Dress with toppings of choice and enjoy.

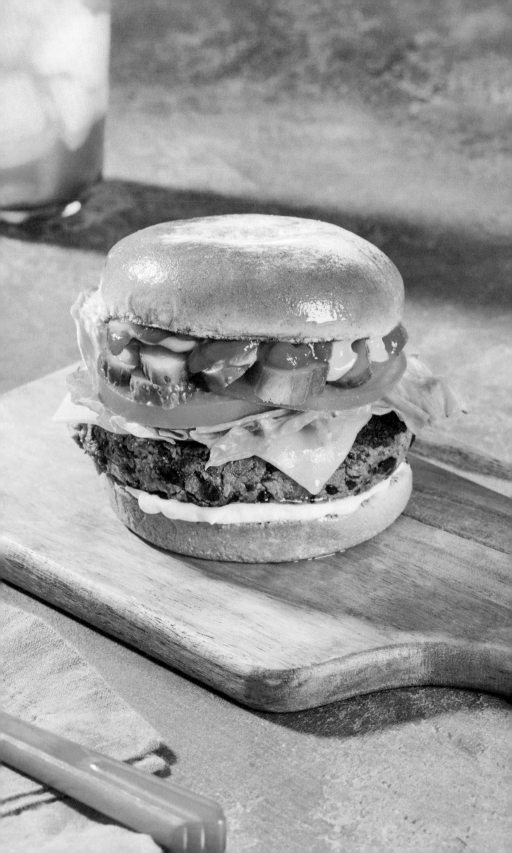

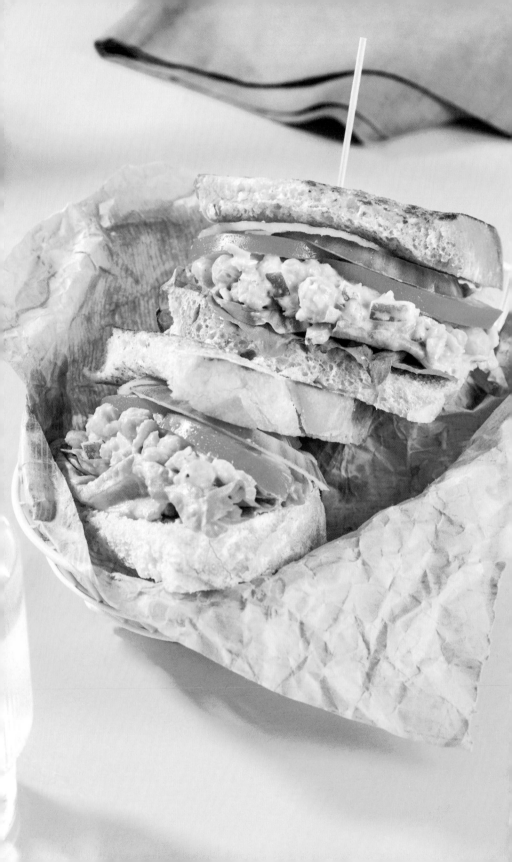

CHICKPEA "TUNA"

Ingredients

3 cups (450 g) cooked chickpeas

½–¾ cup (150 g) vegan mayo

2½ tbsp (37.5 g) relish

¾ cup (112.5 g) red onion, chopped

1 stalk (40 g) celery, chopped

1–1½ tbsp (27 g) salt

1–1½ tbsp (9 g) pepper

1–1½ tbsp (7 g) onion powder

1–1½ tbsp (7 g) garlic powder

juice of half a lemon

Growing up, tuna sandwiches were one of those meals that always were satisfying. The brightness of the lemon and herb notes, the creaminess of the mayo, the acidic hits from the onion and vegetables within made it one of my favorites. All those notes are present but using chickpeas (my favorite legume). Just add everything to a bowl, smash the chickpeas, and it's done.

Instructions

Load ingredients into one mixing bowl. Mix to desired consistency and serve—*easy!*

EASY CAESAR SALAD DRESSING

Ingredients

½ cup (70 g) cashews

3 cloves garlic

1 tbsp (15 g)
Dijon mustard

1 tsp (6) salt

1 tsp (3) pepper

drizzle of olive oil

1 cup (240 g) water

couple inches
of a dill pickle
(approximately 30 g)

Tapped in Wellness

Who have you met that doesn't like a Caesar salad? I know I'm ordering it almost every time I see it on a menu when at a restaurant. The tangy hits combined with a peppery bite all balanced out with a rich and creamy texture all complemented by crisp croutons and romaine. It's a perfect salad. This easy plant-based twist is not a boring, "healthy" version. That same flavor is present and will give you all know about what a Caesar salad has to offer.

Instructions

Load all ingredients into a blender or food processor and blend on high speed until fully homogeneous. Adjust seasonings to taste. Transfer to a sealed container and use as desired.

CROUTONS

Ingredients
3–4 slices bread of choice
drizzle of olive oil
1 tsp (6 g) salt
1 tsp (3 g) pepper
1 tsp (5 g) nutritional yeast
1 tsp (1 g) oregano

Instructions
Cube bread slices and add to a large bowl. Add oil and seasonings and toss to combine. Transfer to a parchment-lined baking sheet and bake at 400°F for 10–15 minutes or until dry and crispy.

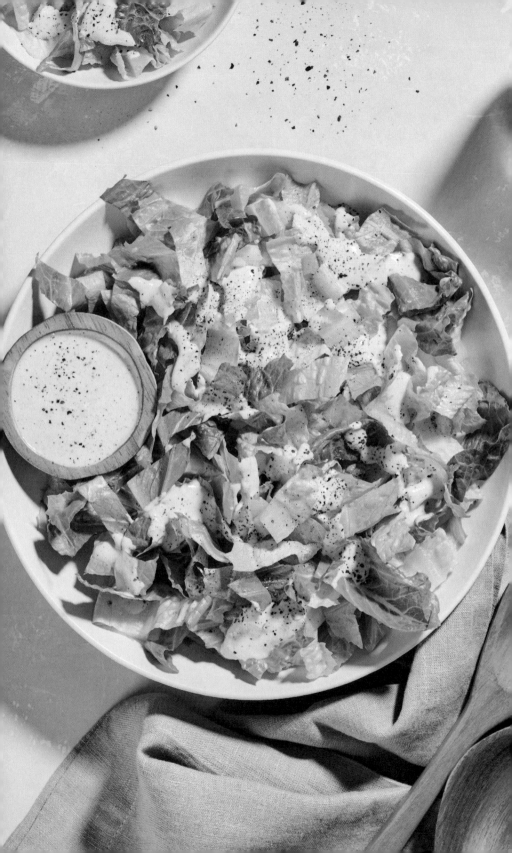

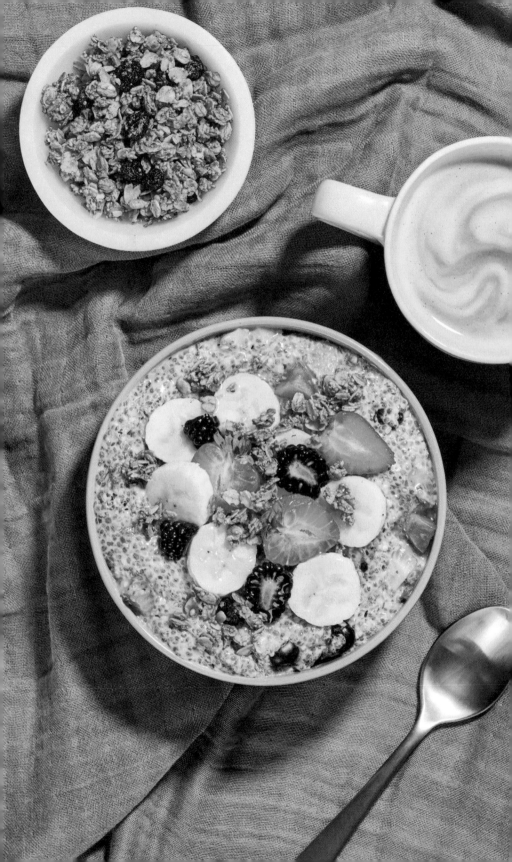

SUPERCHARGED SEED PUDDING

Ingredients

⅓ cup (53 g) chia seeds

⅓ cup (50 g)
  hemp seeds

¼ cup (30 g)
  ground flaxseeds

⅓ cup (55 g)
  strawberry, chopped

3 dates, chopped (24 g)

¼ cup (40 g) dry
  mango, chopped

2-3 cups (480-720 mL)
  plant milk (enough to
  cover mix fully)

When I started my plant-based journey and looked for ways to get nutritious and filling breakfasts, this made me feel I was getting all I needed. The healthy fats and fiber that make up the seeds are a great way to get the brain active and the digestive system started. This is one to prepare overnight but requires minimal effort. Add whatever you like to this to make it your own and play with flavors so you have exciting breakfasts or snacks every day.

Instructions

Add all ingredients to a sealable container or bowl. Pour over plant milk to cover mix fully; it should be runny at this stage. Stir to combine. Cover and place in fridge to thicken, at least 1 hour. Remove from fridge and serve with fruit of choice, granola, plant-based yogurt, or whatever you want!

Section 3: Nutritional Wellness

CHICKPEA FRIED RICE

Ingredients

½ cup (75 g) red pepper, diced

⅓ cup (50 g) scallion, sliced

2 cups (150 g) red cabbage, sliced

⅔ cup (85 g) carrots, sliced

1 thumb of ginger, chopped finely (15 g)

2–3 garlic cloves, chopped finely

1 cup (165 g) cooked chickpeas

2–3 cups (370 to 555 g) cooked rice of choice

1–2 tsp (6–12 g) salt

1–2 tsp (3–6 g) pepper

1–2 tsp (1–2 g) red pepper

1–2 tsp (3–6 g) garlic powder

1–2 tsp (2–4 g) ground coriander

sesame seeds, sliced scallion, lime to garnish

Fried rice is one of those easy and satisfying dishes that can be a vehicle for a lot of nutrition. Being that veggies are a mainstay in a meal like this, it makes it easy to integrate some of your favorites with a lot of flavor in between. Most of the time this dish is in the prep of the veggies but it all comes together in a matter of minutes. Try this chickpea variation for added protein and robust flavors.

Instructions

Slice all veggies and set aside. In a late pan or wok, add all ingredients *except* the rice. Sauté for 2–4 minutes until veggies are soft then add in seasonings and rice. Stir-fry together until all is combined. Taste for seasoning and serve with sesame seeds, scallions, and lime to garnish.

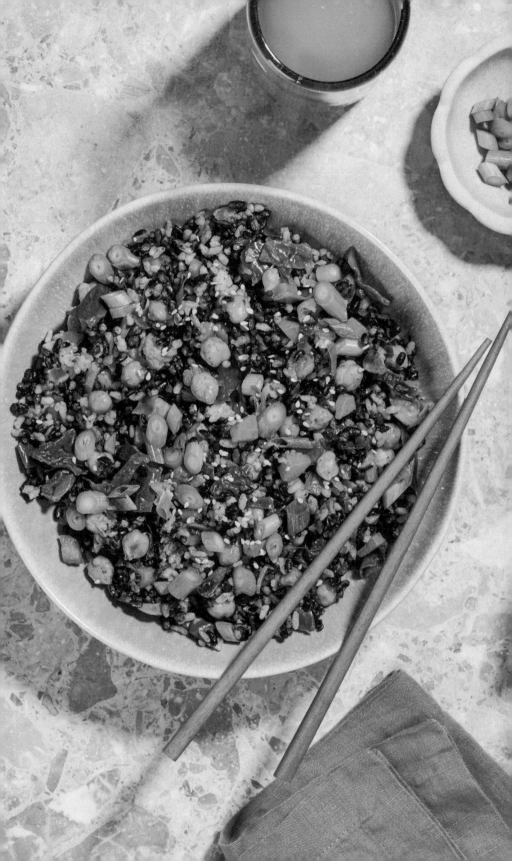

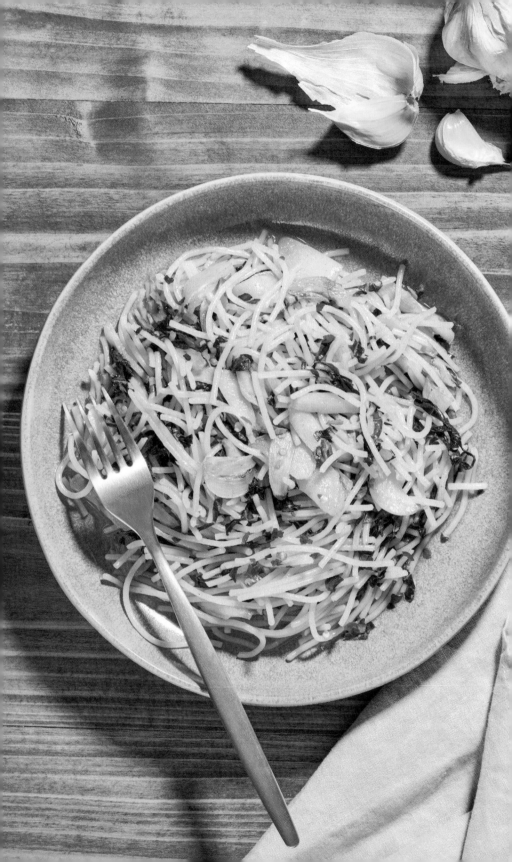

AGLIO E OLIO

Ingredients

8 oz (227 g) spaghetti

1 head garlic, sliced (approximately 40 g)

1 cup (40 g) basil, chopped

½ cup (120 mL) extra virgin olive oil

1 tbsp red chili flakes (15 g) or chili oil (15 mL)

¼ cup (60 mL) pasta water

salt and pepper to taste

squeeze of lemon

I saw this dish in the movie *Chef* and it stuck with me ever since. Once I tried it myself, I understood how simple, in most cases, is better. The quality of a few ingredients can make more of an impression than a host of flavors trying to compete for your attention. The traditional recipe calls for parsley in place of basil but I love basil so much so that's what I suggest you try. Whether you're making this ahead or for a crowd, it's just as easy and just as impactful.

Instructions

Bring pasta to a boil. Meanwhile, peel and slice garlic and chop basil. On a medium-low heat, fry garlic in the olive oil. Once the garlic starts to go slightly brown, add the red chili flakes and turn off the heat. Once pasta is done, add the oil along with the herbs and pasta water and fold together. Salt and pepper to taste, add a squeeze of lemon and extra chili oil or red chili flakes and enjoy.

MAPLE BASIL MUSHROOM TOAST

Ingredients

⅓ cup (13 g) basil, chopped

⅓ cup (80 mL) maple syrup

pinch of salt

1 tsp (2 g) black pepper

1 tsp (3 g) garlic powder

1 tsp (2 g) ground coriander

2 tsp (10 mL) olive oil

2 tsp (9 g) vegan butter

1 medium cluster oyster mushrooms (approximately 100 g)

Maple and basil might seem like an unlikely pairing, but trust me when I say it's one of those combos you'll be wanting to try more. The deep sweetness of the maple syrup coupled with bright and aromatic basil offer a well-rounded flavor profile that go so well with these mushrooms.

Instructions

For the glaze, combine all ingredients (except mushrooms) in a small pan and bring to a simmer for about 5 minutes, then set aside. Peel apart your mushrooms and sauté with a little salt and pepper and optionally press them with another skillet to bring out more of a meaty texture. Once sautéed and crispy, add in the glaze and toss to coat fully. Toast some bread, serve, and enjoy.

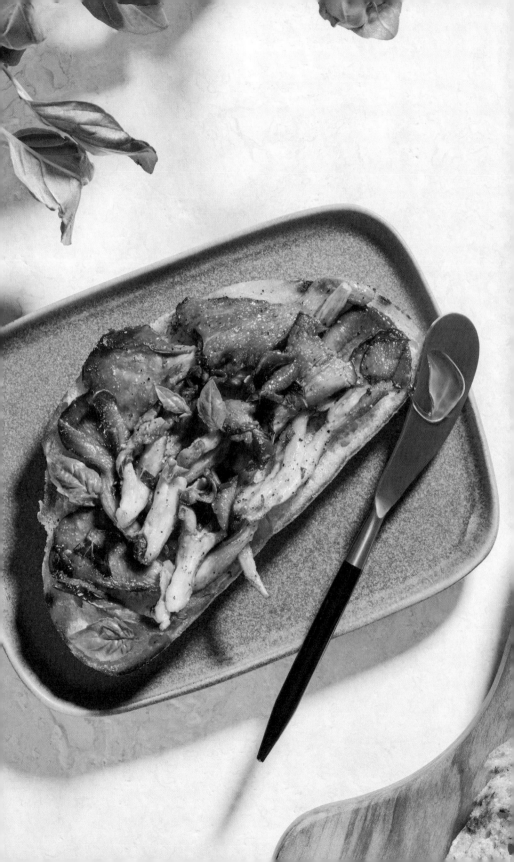

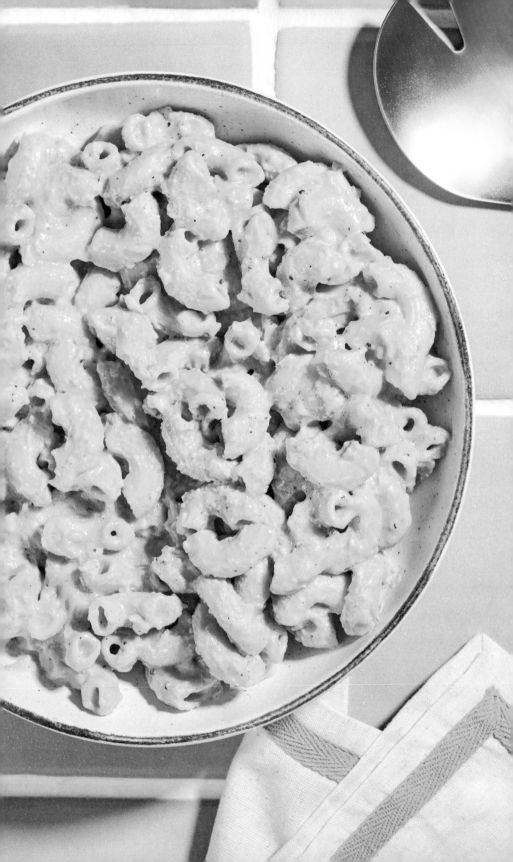

THE BEST VEGAN MAC & "CHEESE"

Ingredients

3 cloves garlic, minced

½ onion, chopped (approximately 70 g)

1⅓ cups (320 mL) unsweetened cashew milk

½ cup (70 g) raw cashews

½ cup (60 g) nutritional yeast

1 can (13.5 oz or 400 mL) full-fat coconut milk

salt and pepper to taste

1 tsp (3 g) turmeric

1 tbsp (14 g) vegan butter

10 oz (283 g) macaroni

I know mac and cheese is one of the dishes vegan cuisine replicates a lot as a means to showcase that you can have it while being plant-based, but I'm going to be real and say most are not that good. The over-the-top replicated cheese flavor and rubbery textures give the dish a bad rap. I like this recipe because it can be made with simple, accessible ingredients and doesn't rely on specialty items that might be harder to find. I wanted to capture the flavors I remember from family gatherings and Mom's mac and cheese. Though she set the standard, let's just say she prefers this one now.

Instructions

Chop garlic and onion. Once prepped, put cashew milk, cashews, and nutritional yeast in a blender and process until combined. Set it aside. Sweat garlic and onion in a separate pan. Once sweated, put in cheese-sauce mixture from blender and coconut milk. Season with salt, pepper, and a little turmeric (for color), and add in vegan butter for a richer flavor and slightly thicker consistency. Simmer until sauce is thick enough to coat the back of a spoon and leave a trail when a finger is run through it. Meanwhile, cook pasta. Once cooked, strain and combine with cheese sauce. Serve and enjoy.

Section 3: Nutritional Wellness

Dishes to Live For

One of the top things I hear about being plant-based, aside from "wHerE dO yOu Get YoUr pRotEin?" is that it is difficult to capture the same flavors and that it just isn't satisfying enough. Coming from a household with Caribbean and Southern American roots, flavor was not lost on me. I knew that transitioning fully to plant-based flavor had to be present along with the nutritional integrity these foods had to offer. These are some of the most satisfying dishes I've developed to date that I think you would love if you tried. Give them a go and see for yourself how amazing plants can be.

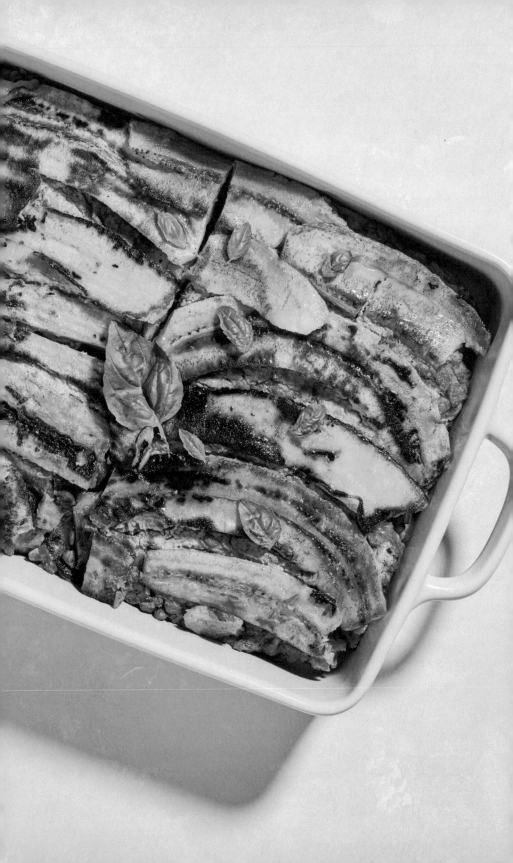

PLANTAIN LASAGNA

Ingredients

⅔ cup (100 g) pumpkin seeds

4 cups (300 g) baby bella mushrooms

1 bell pepper, chopped (approximately 150 g)

½ large onion, chopped (approximately 100 g)

3-4 cloves garlic, minced

8 oz (227 g) cooked brown lentils

3 tbsp (45 mL) coconut aminos

1 can or jar tomato sauce of choice (540 mL or 2¼ cups)

½ cup (40 g) fresh basil, chopped

salt and pepper to taste

10-15 ripe plantains (1,500-2,250 g)

homemade vegan cheese sauce

This is most definitely a top three dish of all time for me. Given my love for plantains I couldn't think of a better way to complement its versatility. I note to use ripe plantains in the written recipe but you could also use some that are slightly more on the unripe side as they offer a different flavor profile that works just as well. The layers of a bright and fragrant tomato sauce with a creamy cheese sauce and caramelized plantain are a combination of flavors that you didn't know you needed in your life.

Instructions

Add the pumpkin seeds and mushrooms to a food processor and pulse until minced fine and resembles coarse sand. Sauté chopped peppers, onion, garlic, and mushroom mix. Then add in the cooked lentils and coconut aminos. Once sautéed, add tomato sauce, seasonings, and basil. Set aside to simmer on low heat. Peel and slice plantains into semi thick strips (should yield about 4 strips per plantain). Parcook the plantains by searing on both sides until golden and set aside. Assemble lasagna by laying down a layer of plantains covering the bottom of the baking dish followed by the tomato sauce and cheese sauce, and repeat 2 or 3 times total. Bake at 355°F for 25 minutes. Let cool and serve.

Cheese Sauce

3 cloves garlic, minced

½ onion, chopped (approximately 70 g)

1⅓ cups (320 mL) plant milk (recommend unsweetened almond or cashew)

½ cup (70 g) cashews

½ cup (60 g) nutritional yeast

1 can (13.5 oz or 400 mL) full-fat coconut milk

salt and pepper to taste

1 tsp (3 g) turmeric (for color, optional)

1 tbsp (14 g) vegan butter (optional)

Prep "Cheese" Sauce: Chop garlic and onion. Add plant milk, cashews, and nutritional yeast to a blender and process until combined. Set aside. Sweat garlic and onion in a separate pan. Strain off blended mixture into the pan and add the coconut milk. Season with salt, pepper, and a little turmeric (for color), and add in vegan butter for a richer flavor and slightly thicker consistency. Simmer until it coats the back of a spoon and leaves a trail when a finger is run through it.

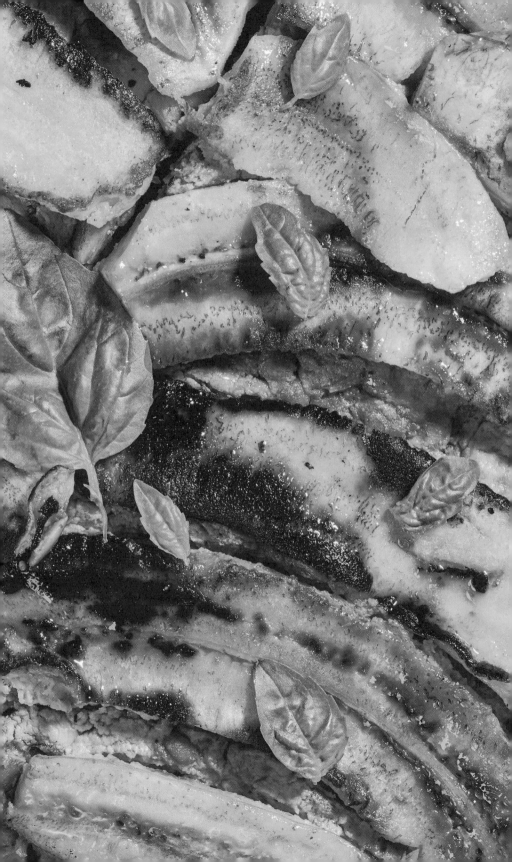

VEGAN "STEAK" DINNER

Ingredients

"Steak"

1 whole lion's
mane mushroom
(150 to 300 g)

salt and pepper

2 tbsp (28 g)
vegan butter

fresh sage and/
or rosemary

Sides

4 mini yellow
potatoes (4oo g)

¼ cup (60 mL) olive oil

3 tsp (18 g) salt

3 tsp (6 g) pepper

3 tsp (9 g) garlic powder

1 bunch of asparagus

The power of mushrooms is infinite. This is another example of how something is prepared can change the eating experience altogether. From the look to the taste and texture, this is one of the dishes that rivals the real thing on its best day. On top of that the benefits of this mushroom are undeniable. Lion's mane is particularly good for brain health and cognition so you get food for your brain and your belly.

Instructions

Preheat oven to 400°F. Boil your potatoes until fork tender. Transfer to a parchment-lined baking sheet and smash with a large glass or other flat surface; drizzle with olive oil; season with salt, pepper, and garlic powder. Roast for 25–30 minutes until golden and crispy. Set aside. Take your whole lion's mane mushroom and set in an oiled cast iron skillet. Let it sit in the pan for 2 minutes, then lay another cast iron skillet on top and press them together to help the mushroom expel moisture. Cook on one side until seared and flip. Season with salt and pepper and press again until you get the size you want. Once seared evenly, place in the 400°F oven for about 10 minutes. Remove from oven, on medium heat, place vegan butter in the pan along with fresh herbs and baste the mushroom. Steam or sauté asparagus with seasonings of choice and serve.

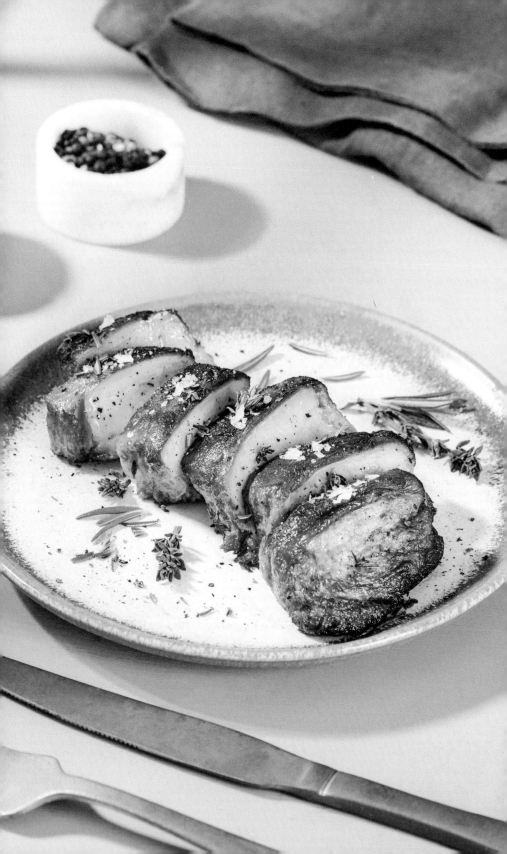

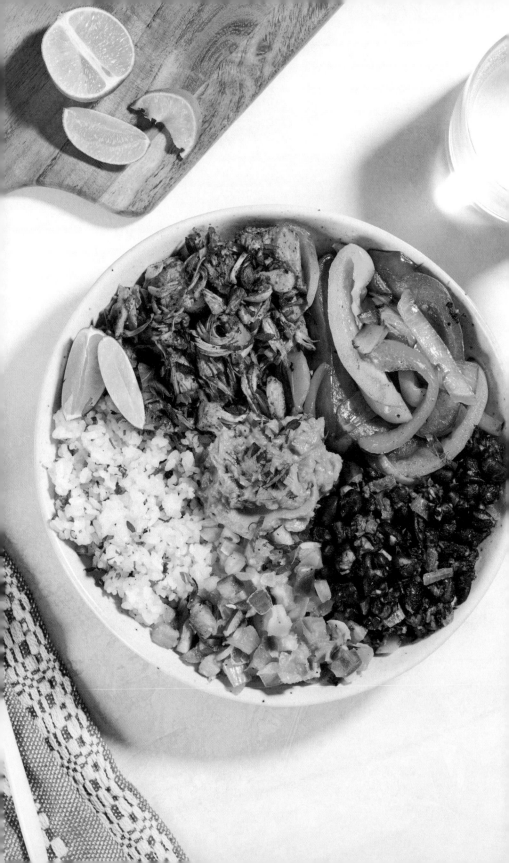

CHIPOTLE-INSPIRED PEPPER JACKFRUIT BOWL

Ingredients

For Rice

⅓ cup of chopped cilantro

Squeeze of half a lime

1 cup rice

For Pepper Jackfruit

2 cans of young green jackfruit (drained and rinsed) (560 g)

4-5 tbsp (60-75 mL) avocado oil

1 tbsp (15 g) garlic, minced

1½ tsp (7.5 g) salt

1½ tsp (3.75 g) onion powder

1½ tsp (3.75 g) smoked paprika

1½ tsp (1.5 g) dried thyme

2 tsp (5.2 g) paprika

2 tsp (4.2 g) crushed chipotle pepper

For Fajita Veggies

¼ red, green, yellow, and orange peppers, sliced (approximately 30 g each)

¼ red onion, sliced lengthwise (approximately 25 g)

For Black Beans

2 cans black beans (drained and rinsed) (560 g)

⅓ cup (79 mL) water

salt and pepper

¼ cup (40 g) red onion, diced

2 tbsp (30 g) garlic, minced

1 tbsp (8 g) chili powder

1 tsp (2.2 g) cumin

For Pico de Gallo

1 large tomato, diced (approximately 180 g)

½ jalapeño, diced (7 g)

⅓ cup (15 g) cilantro, chopped

¼ cup (40 g) red onion, diced

Juice of one lime (or to taste) (approximately 20 mL)

salt and pepper to taste

For Guac

2 avocados (approximately 450 g)

½ cup (80 g) of pico de gallo folded in

salt and pepper to taste

People who go plant-based have cravings and for sure miss some dishes they used to have. But it is more about the memory than the food. The familiarity and experience are what's missed; therefore we can make alternatives to satisfy those cravings. This is one of those for me. This dish is inspired by the flavors from Chipotle, and I wanted to see how I could draw on some of that inspiration to capture a similar experience at home with healthy whole food, plant-based ingredients. Safe to say I think I did that and it's safe to say you should try it too.

Instructions

Cook your rice to package instructions and set aside to cool once done. Drain and rinse your jackfruit; optionally chop the jackfruit into more manageable/bite-sized pieces as they can come quite large. Transfer the drained and rinsed jackfruit to a large bowl and coat in oil, garlic, and spices. Toss to fully coat, cover, and marinate jackfruit for at least 30 minutes. Meanwhile, chop all your peppers and onion for the fajita veggies. Sauté on medium heat with a little oil until slightly charred and soft. Set aside. Add black beans and all other bean ingredients listed in a medium pot and simmer, covered, for 10–15 minutes. While that is going, pan sear the marinated jackfruit until charred and cooked through. For the pico, chop all the ingredients listed and toss together in a bowl like a salad; season to your liking and taste along the way. For the guac, mash avocados in a bowl and add 3–4 tablespoons of your pico de gallo. Fold together and taste for seasoning, adjust to your liking. Assemble your bowl with cilantro lime rice (your cooked rice tossed with lime juice and chopped cilantro) as the base, followed by a layer of the cooked jackfruit, then black beans, fajitas, and some healthy dollops of guac and pico. Enjoy!

Tapped in Wellness

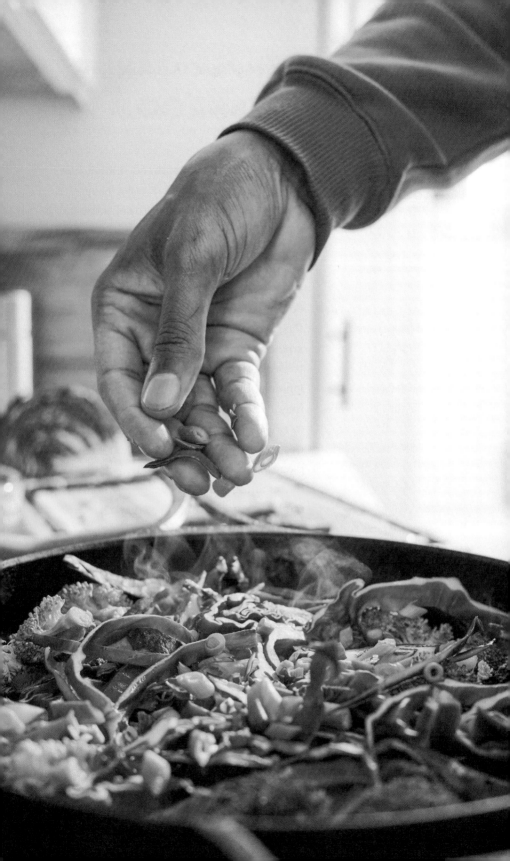

PEPPER GARLIC MUSHROOMS

Ingredients

8 oz (227 g)
oyster mushrooms

For Wet Batter

3 tbsp (21 g)
ground flaxseed

⅓ cup (79 mL) water

2 tbsp (30 mL) sriracha

1 tbsp (15 mL) mustard

2 tbsp (30 mL)
coconut aminos

For Dry Batter

1½ cup (180 g)
chickpea flour

1 tsp (2 g) white pepper

1 tsp (1 g) dried thyme

1 tsp (2 g) paprika

1 tsp (3 g) garlic powder

For Finishing

avocado oil for frying

1 jalapeño
(approximately 14 g)

½ bunch scallions
(approximately 50 g)

5–6 cloves
garlic, chopped

salt and black
pepper to taste

This one is just plain good; I don't know how else to describe it. Notes of salty, spicy, and crispy make this just a great dish, and it is super easy and super satisfying.

Instructions

For the wet batter, combine the ground flax, water, sriracha, mustard, and coconut aminos in a small bowl, mix and set aside to thicken up. Next, combine all dry batter ingredients in a separate bowl, whisk to fully incorporate, and set aside. Separate mushrooms from their cluster into your desired size for consumption. Coat each piece in the wet batter first, then dry batter and repeat that cycle once more until mushrooms are coated fully. Over medium to high heat in a skillet, fry the mushrooms in about two inches of avocado oil until golden and crispy. Set aside. Slice jalapeño and scallion and chop garlic. Sauté over medium heat until fragrant, then add mushrooms, salt, and pepper to taste. Turn off heat and mix to combine. Serve and enjoy.

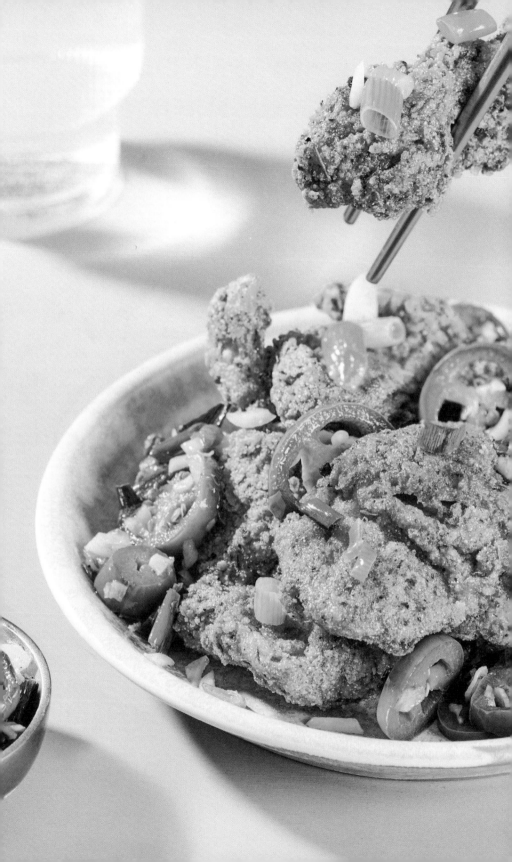

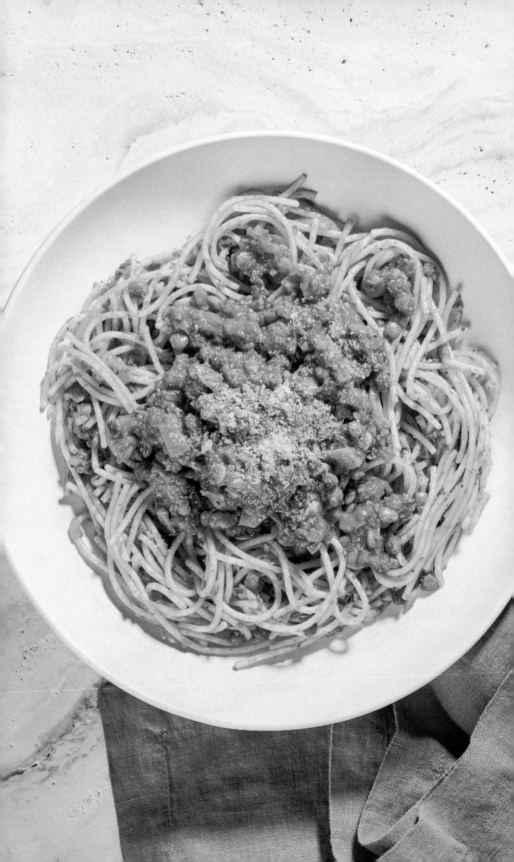

LENTIL BOLOGNESE

Ingredients

1 large yellow onion, chopped (approximately 150 g)

2 medium carrots, chopped (approximately 120 g)

2 stalks celery, chopped (approximately 80 g)

5 cloves garlic, chopped

4 cups (300 g) baby bella mushrooms, chopped

⅔ cup (100 g) pumpkin seeds

3 tbsp (45 mL) coconut aminos

3 tbsp (45 mL) avocado oil

3 tbsp (45 g) tomato paste

2 tsp (4 g) paprika

2 tsp (2 g) dried oregano

2 tsp (2 g) dried basil

2 tbsp (30 mL) balsamic vinegar

salt and pepper to taste

4 cups (900 g) crushed tomatoes

8 oz (227 g) brown lentils

10 oz (283 g) of spaghetti

parsley, chopped, to garnish (approximately 15 g)

vegan parmesan to top

A culinary classic reimagined. I don't think I need to convince you of the place Bolognese holds in the conversation about some of the best foods. I will say that this plant-based version deserves a place in the conversation too. Rich, "meaty," deep flavors cooked into a mushroom- and lentil-based sauce layered over your favorite pasta is enough of a sell for me. Try this and see where it stands for you.

Instructions

Chop carrots, onion, celery, and garlic. (You can also throw all of these into a food processor and pulse until they reach a uniform consistency, be careful not to overdo it here!) Pulse the mushrooms and pumpkin seeds in a food processor until they reach a mostly uniform, crumbly texture. In a large pot sauté the mushroom mixture along with the coconut aminos and avocado oil until most of the moisture has gone. Set aside. In the same pot, add in your chopped carrots, onion, celery, and garlic and sauté until soft. Add in tomato paste and seasonings; cook until fragrant. Add back in the mushrooms along with the balsamic vinegar, crushed tomatoes, and lentils. Reduce heat to low and simmer for at least 20 minutes. Cook your pasta to desired consistency and serve.

Section 3: Nutritional Wellness

LION'S MANE "CHK'N" SANDWICH

Ingredients

1 large lion's mane
mushroom
(approximately
150–300 g)

For Dry Batter

1½ cup (180 g)
chickpea flour

1 tsp (6 g) salt

1 tsp (2 g) pepper

1 tsp (3 g) garlic powder

1 tsp (3 g) onion powder

1 tsp (2 g)
smoked paprika

1 tsp (1 g) dried thyme

1 tsp (1 g) dried parsley

For Wet Batter

5 tbsp (35 g)
ground flaxseeds

¾ cup (177 mL) water

¼ cup (60
mL) hot sauce

1½ tbsp (22.5
mL) mustard

Lion's mane is a mushroom that will truly blow you away. The texture, flavor, and uses it has can make it a great meat replacement that offer so many other health benefits. Using it in this "chicken" sandwich is another way the mushroom continues to impress.

Instructions

Sear the lion's mane in a hot skillet and press it down to release the water content until you reach your desired thickness for the sandwich. Season with salt and pepper lightly. For wet batter, add flaxseeds, water, hot sauce, and mustard. Mix and set aside. For dry batter, add flour and spices, mix, and set aside. Dredge the mushroom in each batter twice. Fry until golden and crispy all around. Let cool on a paper towel–lined plate, assemble sandwich, serve, and enjoy!

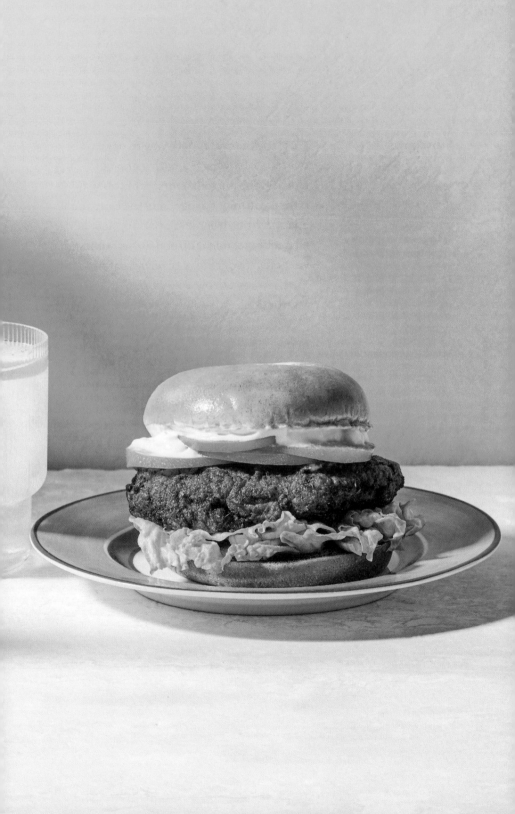

FALAFEL SMASHBURGER

Ingredients

½ white onion (approximately 70 g)

½ large bunch cilantro (approximately 40 g)

½ large bunch parsley (approximately 40 g)

3-4 garlic cloves

1 tbsp (18 g) salt

1 tbsp (6 g) pepper

1 tbsp (8 g) cumin

1 tbsp (5 g) coriander

½-¾ cup (60-90 g) chickpea flour

3 cups (450 g, dry) soaked (uncooked) chickpeas

This is by far my favorite way to have falafel, as if it wasn't amazing enough already. The burger flavors go better with it than you might expect and the light and crispy patties resemble what a typical smashburger might offer. Try this out to find your new favorite way to have falafel.

Instructions

Add all ingredients except chickpea flour into the food processor. Blend to roughly combine, then add in chickpeas and blend again until well combined and fine or transfer to mixing bowl and fold together. Form mix into golf ball-sized portions, add to the pan, smash with a spatula and parchment paper, add your vegan cheese of choice, and assemble with preferred burger toppings.

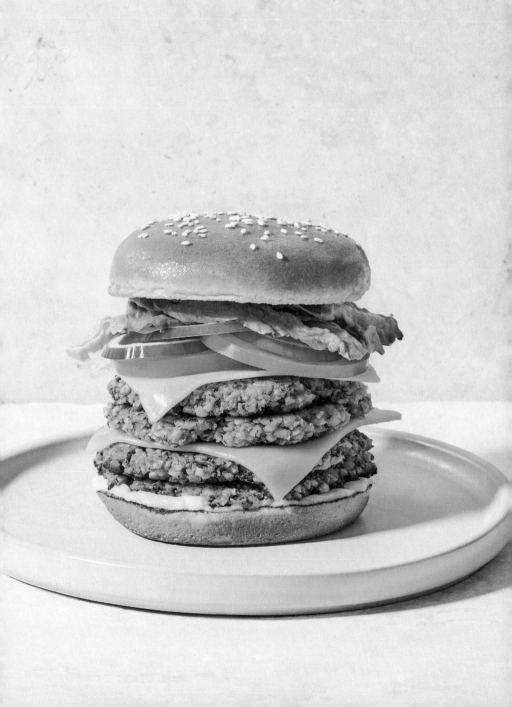

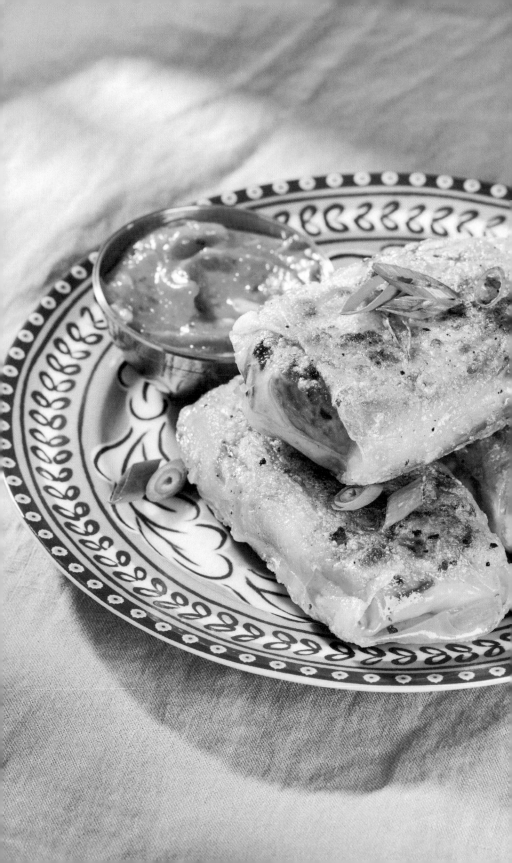

SWEET 'N' SPICY JACKFRUIT SPRING ROLLS

Ingredients

6 rice paper sheets

For Jackfruit

2 8oz cans (454 g) young green jackfruit (drained and rinsed)

3 garlic gloves, grated

1 tbsp (6 g) ginger, grated

1 tbsp (18 g) salt

1 tbsp (6 g) black pepper

1 tbsp (6.8 g) smoked paprika

1 tbsp (7 g) onion powder

3 tbsp (45 mL) maple syrup

1 tbsp (15 mL) chili oil

¼ cup (60 mL) avocado oil

For Peanut Sauce

3 tbsp (48 g) peanut butter

3 tbsp (45 mL) coconut aminos (or soy sauce)

1 tsp (5 mL) sriracha

2 tbsp (30 mL) rice vinegar

1 tbsp (15 mL) lime juice

1 tbsp (15 mL) toasted sesame oil

1 tbsp (15 mL) maple syrup

1 tsp (2 g) ginger

1 tsp (2 g) garlic

I feel like spring rolls have untapped potential. I always feel like they could be filled with something more substantial. So I thought, why not build on that idea and make my dream spring roll? A nice crispy but chewy outer layer, with a rich, umami filling and capped off with a tangy, nutty sauce.

Instructions

Drain and rinse jackfruit and cut into tiny pieces. Marinate for 30 minutes in a bowl along with the ingredients listed above and set aside. Meanwhile make the peanut sauce. Add all ingredients listed above in a bowl and mix until combined. Cook jackfruit in a skillet over medium-high heat until slightly crisp and cooked through. Take your rice paper and fill with about 2–3 tbsp of jackfruit plus any topping you'd like. Double wrap and sear until crisp on both sides. Serve with peanut sauce and enjoy!

ABUNDANT BOWLS— CANNELLINI BEAN BOWL

Tapped in Wellness

Ingredients

For Beans

½ of a shallot, chopped (approximately 20 g)

6 cloves garlic, sliced

½ green bell pepper, chopped (approximately 75 g)

1 can (439 g) cannellini beans (drain half of the liquid)

1 tbsp (15 g) tomato paste

¼ cup (60 mL) coconut milk

1 tsp (6 g) salt

1 tsp (2 g) pepper

For Potato Wedges

4 baby yellow potatoes (approximately 400 g)

1 tsp (6 g) salt

1 tsp (2 g) pepper

1 tsp (3 g) garlic powder

1 tsp (1 g) dried thyme

1 tsp (1 g) dried basil

Vegetables

2 small bok choy (approximately 250 g)

1 cup (90 g) broccoli

Instructions

Chop your shallot, garlic, and green pepper, and sauté in a medium saucepan until softened and fragrant. To the same saucepan, add the beans, tomato paste, coconut milk, and spices listed. Simmer for 2–3 minutes or until it slightly thickens. For potato wedges, chop the potatoes and coat in oil and spices listed. Air fry at 380°F for 25 minutes. Steam bok choy and broccoli in a small skillet over high heat with about a half inch of water; cover with a lid. Remove the veggies once they are bright green and fork tender, add them to complete bowl, and enjoy.

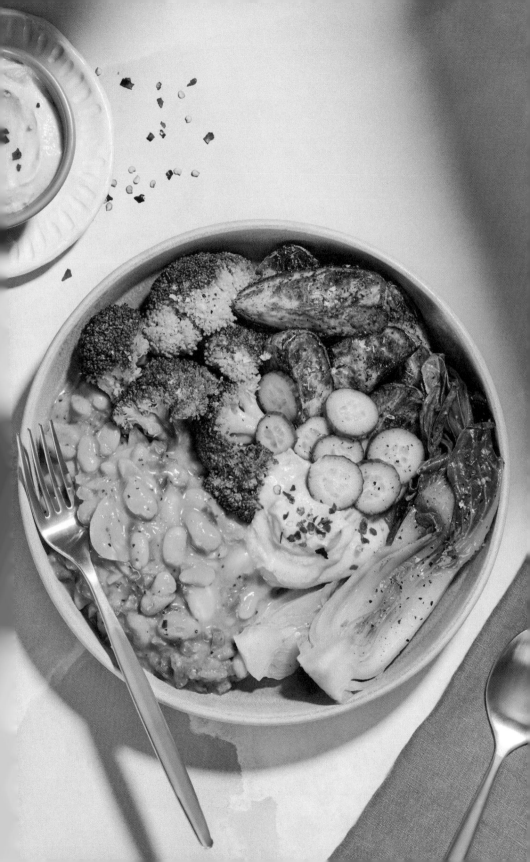

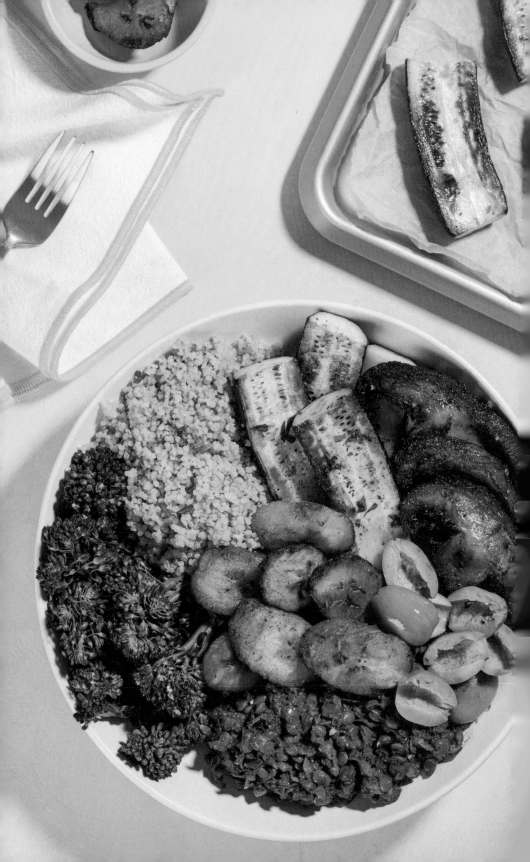

ABUNDANT BOWLS—JERK LENTIL BOWL

Ingredients

For Quinoa

1 cup (170 g) quinoa

1 cup (240 mL) coconut milk

2 bay leaves

1 veggie stock seasoning cube

1½ cup (360 mL) water

For Mushrooms

2 portobello caps, sliced (approximately 120 g)

oil to coat (approximately 15 mL)

1½ tsp (9 g) salt

1½ tsp (3 g) pepper

2 tbsp (14 g) smoked paprika

1½ tsp (4.5 g) garlic and onion powder

1 tsp (1 g) dried basil

For Lentils

½ shallot, chopped (approximately 20 g)

½ red bell pepper, chopped (approximately 75 g)

4 cloves garlic, chopped

1 scallion, chopped (approximately 15 g)

1 tsp (2 g) ginger, chopped

1 can (400 g) lentils (drained and rinsed)

½ cup (120 g) tomato sauce

1 tsp (6 g) salt

1 tsp (2 g) pepper

1 tsp (3 g) garlic powder

1 tsp (3 g) onion powder

1 tsp (1 g) dried thyme

2 tsp (4 g) allspice

½ tsp (1 g) cinnamon

½ tsp (1 g) cayenne

1 tbsp (15 mL) browning (can use soy sauce or coconut aminos)

For Vegetables

1 small bunch of broccolini (approximately 200 g)

1 green zucchini (approximately 200 g)

Pinch of salt and pepper

Instructions

Cook quinoa by adding all ingredients listed to a medium pot. Bring the mix up to a boil; once it reaches a boil, turn the heat down to low and let it simmer for 15 minutes or until all the liquid is absorbed. Turn off heat, and let it steam for 10 minutes covered. Then fluff with a fork and serve. Drain and rinse your lentils. Set aside. Then chop your shallot, bell pepper, scallion, garlic, and ginger and sauté in a medium saucepan with 2 tablespoons of avocado oil until fragrant and soft. Then add in the drained and rinsed lentils, tomato sauce, jerk spices listed, and browning (or soy sauce or coconut aminos). Cover and simmer for 5–8 minutes on medium low heat. For mushrooms, toss in a bowl with oil and spices listed to coat, then air fry at 375°F for 15 minutes. Finally steam the vegetables in a small skillet over high heat with a about a half inch of water; cover with a lid. Remove the veggies once they are bright green and fork tender, and season lightly with salt and pepper. Assemble bowl and enjoy.

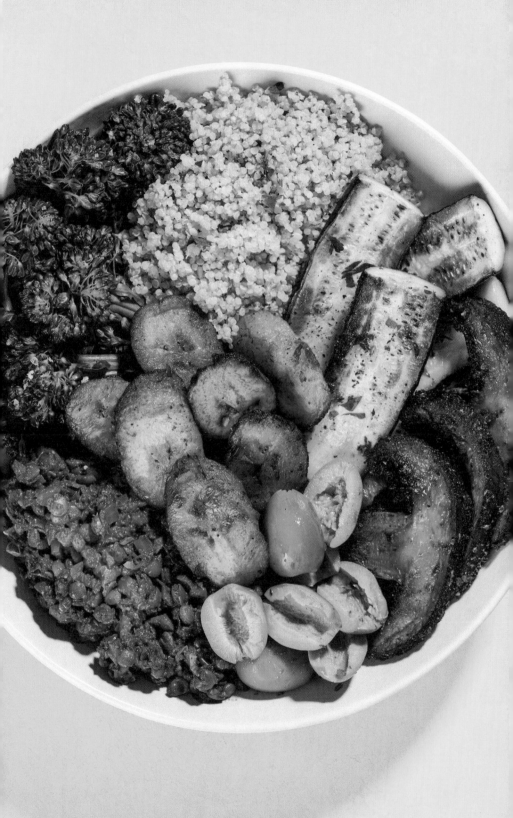

Soulful Sweets

Sweets and desserts are often met with an attitude of guilt or restraint; they feel like something you have to earn or can only enjoy once you have justified it by some other means. It does not have to be this way. Sweets can be enjoyed freely and a few simple swaps in ingredients can change the nutritional value, glycemic index, gluten content that make it indulgent and clean. Get into these dishes and feel the difference for yourself.

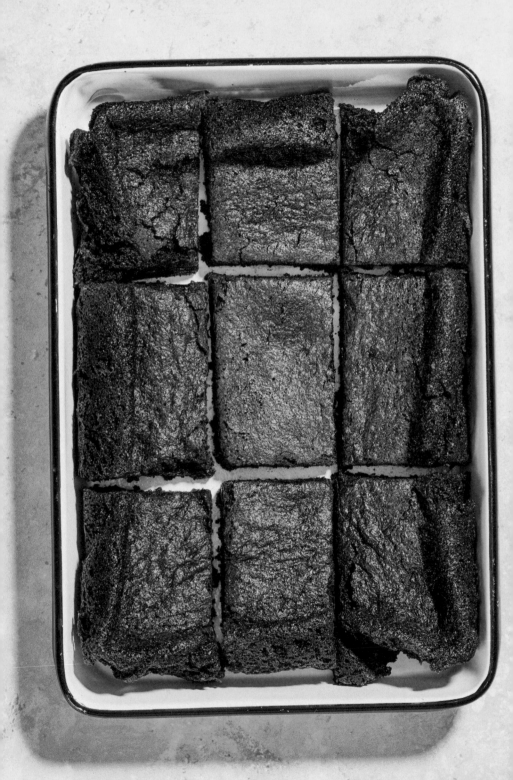

NOT YOUR BASIC BROWNIES (GF)

Ingredients

1 tbsp (10 g) chia seeds

3 tbsp (45 mL) water

1½ cups (300 g) organic cane sugar

¾ cup (180 mL) melted coconut oil

½ cup (120 mL) nondairy milk of choice

1 tsp (5 mL) maple syrup or vanilla extract

1¾ cup (210 g) chickpea flour

½ cup (50 g) cacao powder

1 tsp (4 g) baking soda

When done right, brownies are one of the best sweets to have. And I know there are split sides on this, but my personal favorite way to have them is when the top and crust are crispy and the inside is chewy and gooey. The two textures make for a beautiful combination and an undeniable dessert.

Instructions

Mix chia seeds and water and set aside to thicken. Preheat oven to 375°F. Combine sugar, oil, nondairy milk, and maple syrup/vanilla extract in a bowl until homogenous. Once combined, add in flour, cacao powder, and baking soda, along with chia seed "egg." Mix all together. Pour combined batter into parchment-lined baking pan and distribute evenly. Bake for 28 minutes and let cool.

Section 3: Nutritional Wellness

SIMPLE SNICKERDOODLES

Ingredients

- ½ cup (113 g) vegan butter
- 1 cup (200 g) sugar
- ¼ cup (60 mL) plant milk of choice
- 1 teaspoon (5 mL) vanilla
- 2 cups (240 g) chickpea flour
- 1½ tsp (6 g) baking powder
- ¼ cup (50 g) sugar
- 3 tsp (6 g) cinnamon

When initially going plant-based, I had a mental list of all my favorite foods I wanted to know how to make vegan and this was on that list as this is my favorite cookie. Learning how to make this also taught me that plant-based cooking isn't as difficult as it is perceived to be. A few key replacements and you have something that's just as you know it to be.

Instructions

Preheat oven to 350°F. In a large mixing bowl, add vegan butter and sugar. Mix until creamy and combined. Then add plant milk and vanilla and mix all together. Once wet mix is combined, add in flour and baking powder and mix until dough forms. Once formed, take out dough and roll up golf ball–sized pieces. Coat dough in cinnamon and sugar mix. Line on parchment paper–lined baking sheet and bake at 350°F for 10–15 minutes. Let cool and enjoy!

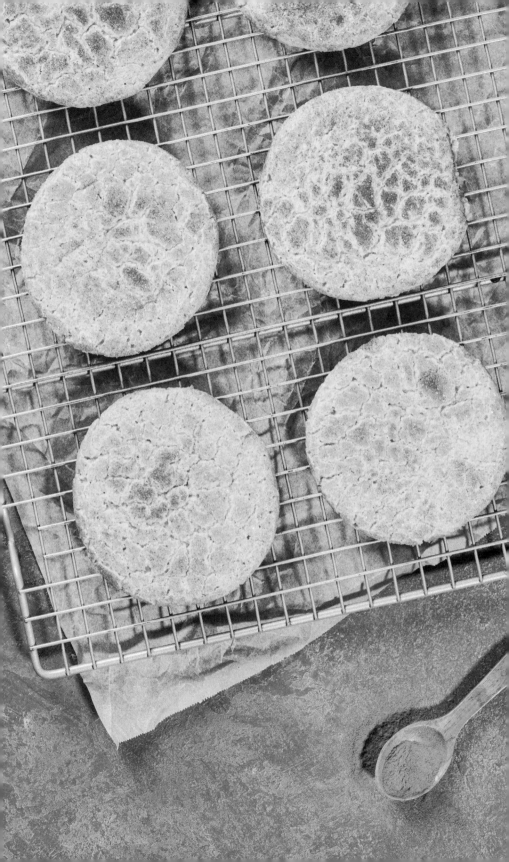

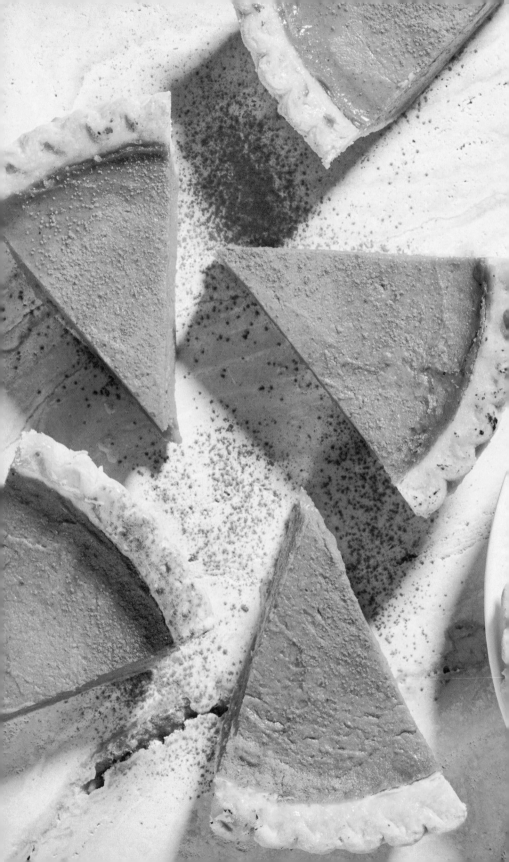

SWEET POTATO PIE

Ingredients

For Crust

2¼ cup (280 g) all-purpose flour

½ cup (113 g) vegan butter or coconut oil

1 tsp (6 g) salt

1 tbsp (12 g) sugar

½ cup (120 mL) ice water

For Filling

2 large boiled, peeled, and mashed sweet potatoes (approximately 500 g)

¼ cup (50 g) coconut sugar

¼ cup (55 g) brown sugar

1½ tbsp (14 g) cinnamon

¼ tsp (0.5 g) nutmeg

1 can (400 mL) coconut milk

3 tbsp (27 g) arrowroot starch

This dish reminds me of all the family gatherings and holidays where my family members would bring all the dishes they were known for. I always looked forward to my aunt's sweet potato pie. The recipe, which was originally my great-grandmother's, wasn't too far off from what you see here. Minus the dairy ingredients, the integrity of the recipe is well intact and approved by the family matriarchs themselves.

Instructions

Crust

Add flour, sugar, and salt to food processor, pulse to combine. Once combined, add vegan butter or coconut oil and pulse until mixture is crumbly and resembles wet sand. Stream in the ice water while blending until rough dough forms. Turn out onto a floured work surface and knead until dough fully forms and shape into a ball. Roll out the dough large enough to cover your pie pan. Shape the dough to the pan, cut the excess off the sides, crimp the edges, and set aside until ready to use.

Filling

Add all ingredients to a blender and blend until homogeneous. Once combined, add to the raw crust. Bake at 350°F for 50–60 minutes. Let cool and refrigerate overnight to fully set. Once set, serve and enjoy.

APPLE CRISP

Ingredients

For Filling

2 lbs apples
(about 4-5 total,
approximately 900 g)

1 tsp (2 g) lemon zest

1 tsp (2 g) orange zest

1½ tbsp (22 mL)
lemon juice

1½ tbsp (2 mL)
orange juice

¼ cup (50 g)
coconut sugar

1 tbsp (8 g)
chickpea flour

1-2 tbsp
(8-16 g) cinnamon

¼ tsp (0.5 g) nutmeg

For Topping

1 cup (120 g) flour

⅓ cup (67 g)
coconut sugar

⅓ cup (73 g) brown
sugar (sticky)

1 cup (90 g) oats

8 tbsp (113 g) vegan
butter (cold)

If you asked me what my favorite dessert was, this would have to be it. The crispy and buttery topping with a gooey and sweet filling is a perfect match in my opinion. There isn't a time or occasion I wouldn't recommend making this.

Instructions

Preheat oven to 350°F. Peel and chop apples, put in a bowl along with zest, juice, sugar, flour, cinnamon, and nutmeg. Toss until apples are evenly coated. Add to your baking dish. In a mixer or medium mixing bowl add sugar, oats, flour, and butter. Mix until coarse and crumbly. Top in your baking over the apples evenly. Bake for 50 minutes. Let cool, serve, and enjoy!

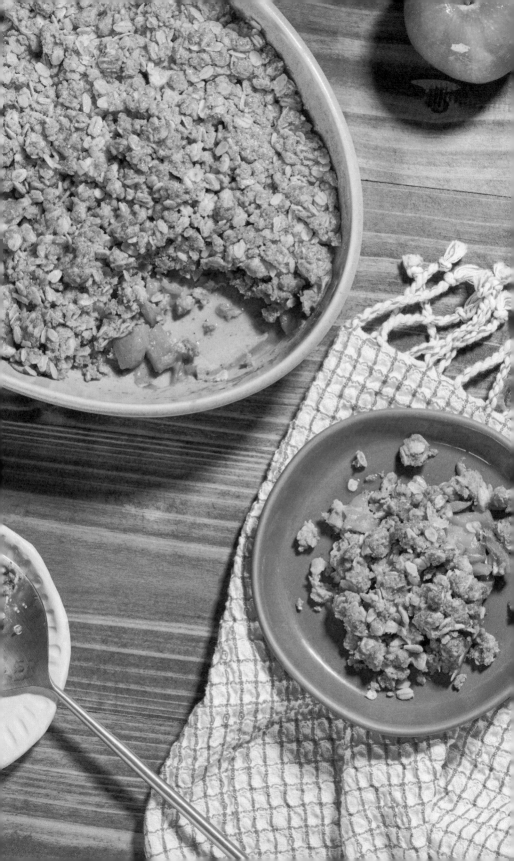

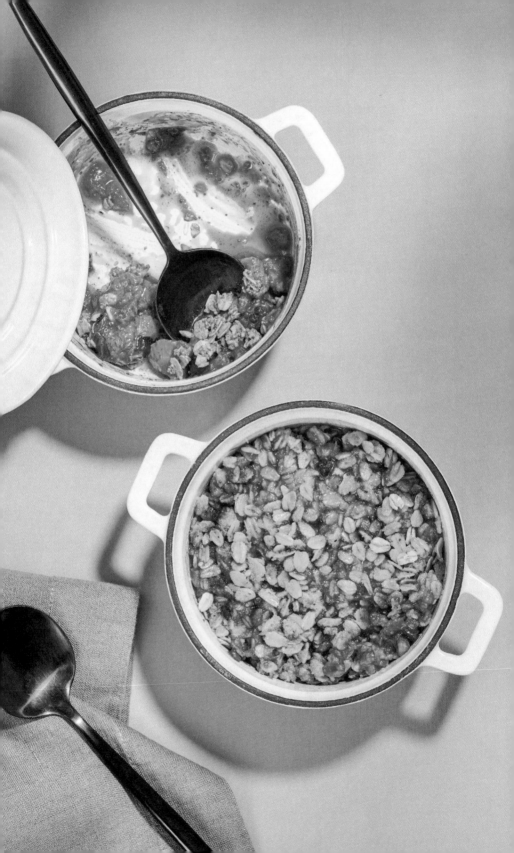

SINGLE-SERVE BERRY CRISP (GF)

A good crisp is my favorite dessert but sometimes a whole one can be more than you might want at a time. Enter the single-serve crisp, berry edition. Make this when you have your next crisp craving.

Ingredients

For Filling

1½ cups (225 g) berries of choice

1 tbsp (12 g) coconut sugar

½ tsp (2 g) arrowroot powder

1 tbsp (15 mL) lemon juice

For Topping

2 tbsp (30 mL) melted vegan butter or coconut oil

2 tbsp (24 g) brown sugar

2 tbsp (14 g) almond flour

4 tbsp (24 g) gluten-free oats

Instructions

Preheat your oven to 350°F. Add your berries, sugar, arrowroot powder, and lemon juice into a small heatproof bowl and mix until berries are evenly coated. Set aside. Melt the vegan butter or coconut oil in a small bowl and add the sugar, flour, and oats. Mix to combine. Once mixed, add the crumble on top of the berry mixture and cover evenly. Then place in the oven and bake for 35–40 minutes. Let cool and enjoy.

Section 3: Nutritional Wellness

OATMEAL CRANBERRY RAISIN COOKIES (GF)

Ingredients

- ½ cup (113 g) vegan butter or solidified coconut oil
- 1 cup (200 g) coconut sugar
- ¼ cup (60 mL) plant milk
- ¾ cup (90 g) chickpea flour
- 1 tbsp (8 g) cinnamon
- 1½ tsp (6 g) baking powder
- ¾ cup (60 g) gluten-free rolled oats
- ¼ cup (30 g) dried cranberry
- ¼ cup (40 g) raisins

Oatmeal raisin cookies get unnecessary slander, in my opinion. Where it comes from, I couldn't tell you. I do know oatmeal cookies need more respect for their name, hence this recipe. Adding the cranberries gives a tarter note that contrasts with the raisins within that would put the oatmeal cookie in a better light.

Instructions

Preheat oven to 350°F. To a large mixing bowl add the vegan butter and sugar. Mix until combined into a smooth, thick, paste-like consistency. Add plant milk and mix to combine. Once mixed, add flour, cinnamon, baking powder, and oats on top of the wet mixture and stir on top of the wet mix a few times to roughly combine the dry ingredients before fully mixing both batters together. From here the cookie dough should form. Once dough starts to form, add in the cranberries and raisins and fold into the dough. Use an ice cream scoop to scoop out dough onto a parchment-lined baking pan. Slightly pat down each scoop on the pan and bake for 20–25 minutes or until slightly golden. Let cool and enjoy.

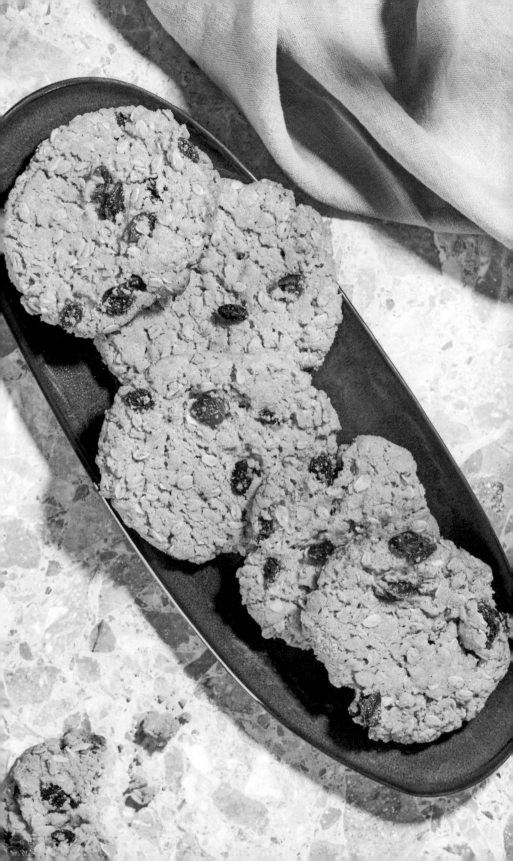

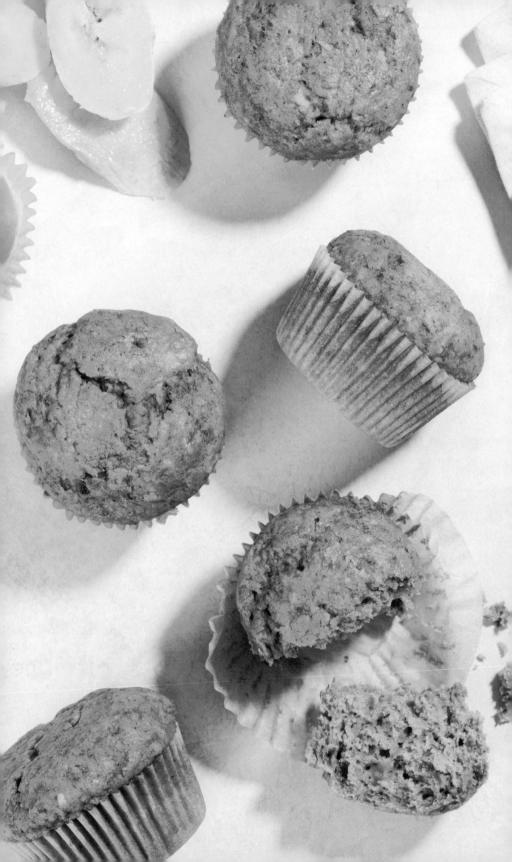

SPICED PLANTAIN MUFFINS

Ingredients

- 1½ cups (180 g) organic all-purpose flour
- 1 tsp (4 g) baking powder
- 1 tsp (4 g) baking soda
- 1 tsp (2 g) cinnamon
- ½ tsp (1 g) allspice
- ¼ tsp (0.5 g) nutmeg
- 1 large very ripe plantain (approximately 200 g)
- ¾ cup (150 g) coconut sugar
- ¾ to 1 cup (180–250 mL) plant milk
- ⅓ cup (160 mL) melted vegan butter or coconut oil

The Caribbean in me had to question what a muffin would be like with a plantain instead of a banana, not too farfetched of an idea. I found the plantain offers a deeper, more robust flavor as opposed to a lighter and fruitier flavor from a banana. The spices give a warm and comforting essence that is perfect for a cozy night in or a chilly day.

Instructions

Preheat oven to 375°F. In a large mixing bowl, add flour, baking powder, baking soda, and spices. Whisk, then set aside. Mash the plantain in a separate bowl, then add sugar, plant milk, and melted vegan butter or coconut oil. Mix until incorporated. Add both wet and dry mixes together until batter forms. Line muffin tray with baking cups. Scoop out batter and distribute evenly into the tray. Bake for 20–25 minutes. Let cool and enjoy!

NO-BAKE MINI CARROT CAKES (GF)

Ingredients

For Crust

1 cup (175 g)
medjool dates

1 cup (100 g)
raw walnuts

1 tbsp (8 g) cinnamon

1 cup (110 g)
shredded carrots

pinch of salt

For Filling

½ cup (120 mL)
coconut cream

⅓ cup (67 g)
coconut sugar

4 tbsp (60 mL)
lemon juice

1 tsp (5 mL)
vanilla extract

⅔ cup (160 g) vegan
cream cheese

½ cup almond flour
(48 g) or coconut
flour (60 g)

3 tbsp (24 g)
arrowroot starch

Sometimes we want a sweet treat but can't be bothered to turn the oven on. If that's you, this is the treat to go for. They come together quickly, no cooking is involved, and they're easy to store in the fridge or freezer to enjoy later.

Instructions

Line a muffin tin with baking cups and set aside. In a blender or food processor, add in the dates and blend until roughly processed and still chunky. Remove dates from blender, add in walnuts, cinnamon, carrots, and salt. Blend until roughly combined, then add back in the dates and pulse few more times to get everything mixed together. Spoon mixture into muffin tin and pat down until packed tightly. In a blender add in all filling ingredients and blend until smooth. Pour mixture on top of each crust portion to cover completely. Once all cakes have been poured, tap the tin on your counter to knock out all air bubbles and even out the mix. Set in freezer or fridge to set completely before serving (at least 2–4 hours). Let thaw partially before consumption.

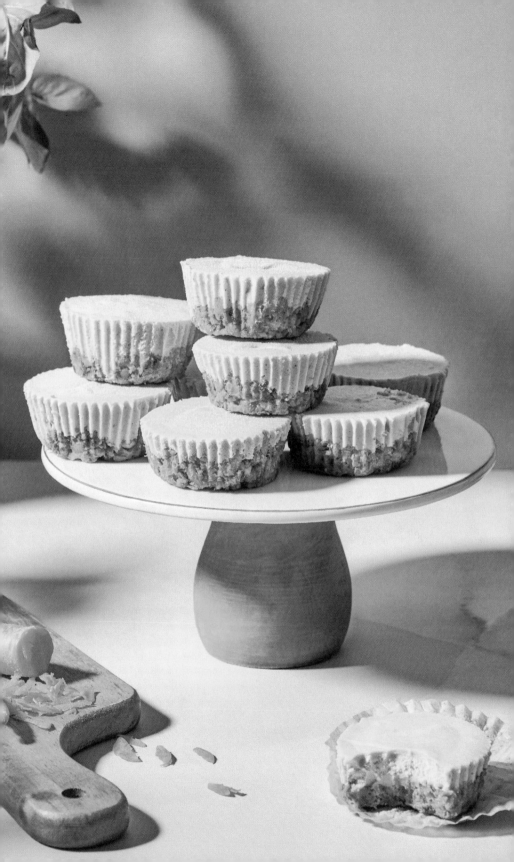

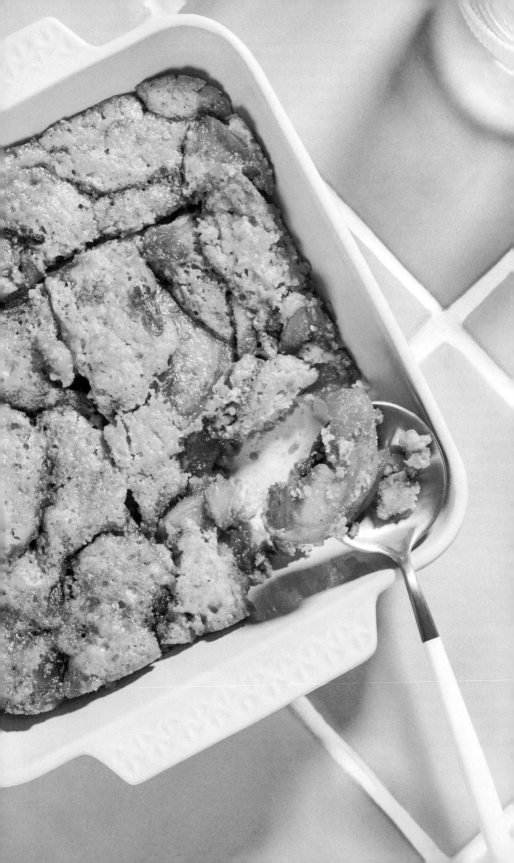

Ingredients

For Filling

5 fresh peaches (about 4 cups, 600 g)

⅔ cup (133 g) coconut sugar

¼ tsp (1.5 g) salt

For Crust

1 cup (120 g) all-purpose flour (can be swapped for GF)

¾ cup (150 g) brown sugar (can sub with coconut sugar)

1 tbsp (14 g) baking powder

¼ tsp (1.5 g) salt

2 tbsp (30 mL) maple syrup

1 tsp (5 mL) vanilla extract

½ cup (120 mL) plant milk

½ cup (120 mL) melted vegan butter

2 tsp (4 g) cinnamon

You can't go wrong with a classic like peach cobbler, and why not have a plant-based version in your repertoire? This Southern staple can be enjoyed any time but hits different when peaches are in season in the summer months.

Instructions

Preheat oven to 350°F. Peel the peaches. Cut them in half and slice into equal-sized pieces. In a large skillet, add the peaches, sugar, and salt over medium heat. Stir and cook for about 5 minutes until slightly tender. Remove and set aside. In a mixing bowl, add the flour, brown sugar, baking powder, and salt. Whisk together. Then add the maple syrup, vanilla, and plant milk. Stir to combine until batter forms, but be careful not to overmix; it's okay if slightly lumpy. Pour the melted butter into the bottom of a baking dish and spread to make an even layer. Pour the batter into the dish over the butter and gently spread but don't mix. Pour the cooked peaches and juice over top of the mixture. Sprinkle with ground cinnamon on top. Bake for 35–45 minutes. Let cool and serve.

Section 3: Nutritional Wellness

FRESH BERRIES AND CREAM

Ingredients

For Berries

1 cup (150 g) strawberries

1 cup (150 g) blueberries

1 cup (140 g) blackberries

1 cup (125 g) raspberries

⅓ cup (67 g) coconut sugar

squeeze of lemon (approximately 5 mL)

2 tbsp (5.6 g) mint, chopped

For Cream

1 cup (240 mL) coconut cream

2 tbsp (24 g) coconut sugar

splash of vanilla extract (approximately 5 mL)

3 tbsp (45 mL) plant-based yogurt

There's power in simplicity and this dish is just that. Juicy berries, creamy topping, and mint make for a light and fresh treat that can be enjoyed at any time and can be made with a myriad of fruits.

Instructions

Add your berries to a large mixing bowl along with the coconut sugar. Squeeze the lemon in, chop your mint, add to berries, and fold together with a spatula. Set aside. Meanwhile, in another bowl, add the coconut cream along with coconut sugar and vanilla extract. Whip with a hand mixer or whisk vigorously by hand until fluffy and peaks form. Add in the plant-based yogurt and gently fold in. Assemble dish with a layer of berries followed by cream, optionally dust cinnamon, and extra mint leaves to garnish.

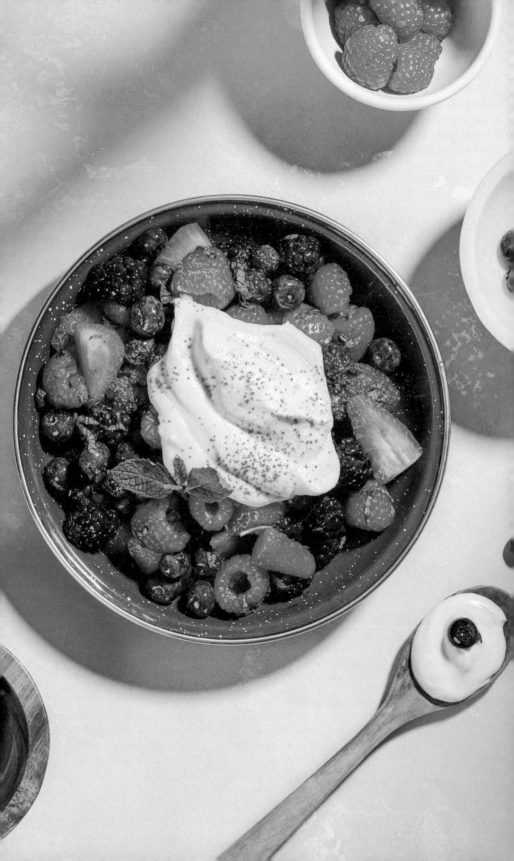

WELLNESS TRACKER

We've gone over a lot in this book so far, and maybe you're thinking about how you might be able to actionably implement some of what you picked up along the way...or at least how to take that first step in a new direction. On the following pages, you'll find your personal Wellness Tracker. This should serve as a small entry point, or another tool, in your journey to help further your wellness goals. There are three sections corresponding with each of the pillars we went over through the book, Mental, Physical and Nutritional Wellness. In each of the sections, you could enter small "wellness wins" from your day. A good place to start would be to jot down bullet points of what you did for yourself in each area and how each made you feel, what it brought up, and/or how you can build from it.

Mental

-
-
-

Nutritional

-
-
-

Physical

-
-
-

Mental

-
-
-

Nutritional

-
-
-

Physical

-
-
-

Mental

_____

_____

_____

_____

_____

_____

Nutritional

_____

_____

_____

_____

_____

_____

Physical

_____

_____

_____

_____

_____

_____

Mental

-
-
-

Nutritional

-
-
-

Physical

-
-
-

Mental

-
-
-

Nutritional

-
-
-

Physical

-
-
-

Mental

-
-
-

Nutritional

-
-
-

Physical

-
-
-

Mental

Nutritional

Physical

Mental

-
-
-

Nutritional

-
-
-

Physical

-
-
-

Mental

Nutritional

Physical

Mental

-
-
-

Nutritional

-
-
-

Physical

-
-
-

Mental

Nutritional

Physical

Mental

-
-
-

Nutritional

-
-
-

Physical

-
-
-

Mental

Nutritional

Physical

Mental

-
-
-

Nutritional

-
-
-

Physical

-
-
-

Mental

Nutritional

Physical

Mental

-
-
-

Nutritional

-
-
-

Physical

-
-
-

Mental

Nutritional

Physical

Mental

-
-
-

Nutritional

-
-
-

Physical

-
-
-

Mental

Nutritional

Physical

Mental

-
-
-

Nutritional

-
-
-

Physical

-
-
-

Mental

Nutritional

Physical

Mental

-
-
-

Nutritional

-
-
-

Physical

-
-
-

Mental

Nutritional

Physical

Mental

-
-
-

Nutritional

-
-
-

Physical

-
-
-

Mental

_____
_____
_____
_____
_____
_____
_____

Nutritional

_____
_____
_____
_____
_____
_____
_____

Physical

_____
_____
_____
_____
_____
_____
_____

Mental

-
-
-

Nutritional

-
-
-

Physical

-
-
-

Mental

-
-
-

Nutritional

-
-
-

Physical

-
-
-

Mental

-
-
-

Nutritional

-
-
-

Physical

-
-
-

Mental

Nutritional

Physical

Mental

-
-
-

Nutritional

-
-
-

Physical

-
-
-

Mental

Nutritional

Physical

Mental

-
-
-

Nutritional

-
-
-

Physical

-
-
-

Mental

Nutritional

Physical

Mental

-
-
-

Nutritional

-
-
-

Physical

-
-
-

Mental

-
-
-

Nutritional

-
-
-

Physical

-
-
-

Mental

-
-
-

Nutritional

-
-
-

Physical

-
-
-

Mental

-
-
-

Nutritional

-
-
-

Physical

-
-
-

Mental

-
-
-

Nutritional

-
-
-

Physical

-
-
-

Mental

Nutritional

Physical

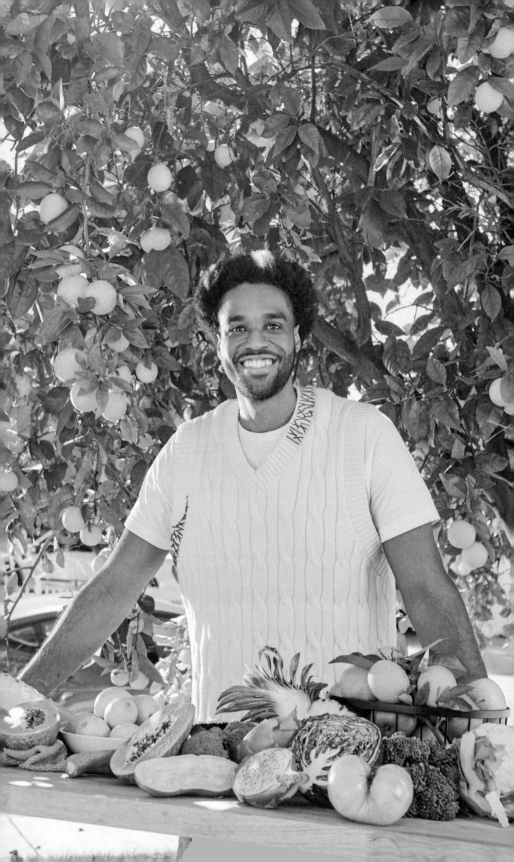

Conclusion

There is so much power in taking steps toward a better life for you. I know through things I have experienced that walking that path, while sometimes uncomfortable, is one of the most gratifying feelings there is. As habits start to stick, as your body starts to change, as your mind begins to sharpen, there is an undeniable shift within that you cannot look back on. Once you know it, feel it, and experience it, it is impossible to unsee it. That is what I wish for you: for your life practices to positively impact you so profoundly that you will not revert to what once was. This doesn't mean all of what was done before was bad; it's all about evolution. Continuing to grow, expand, and learn is what this journey is all about.

We've all been at a point where we knew we desired something greater, something deeper for ourselves and it takes courage to step out into the unknown to find it but I hope you can if you haven't already. If you have, great, you'll probably have to do it again at some point. Tap into the capacity you have within. Align with what lights up your soul. Surround yourself with all the tools necessary for you to succeed in the way you envision. Along the way, enjoy the process even though it seems mundane or slow. Fall into it fully; you will be met with all you need to get to where you want and then some.

These three pillars of mental and spiritual, physical, and nutritional health all fold into the holistic picture that is your wellness. Take time to look into each area and fine-tune them to fit your goals. Maybe some of what has been laid out in this book resonates and maybe some don't, and that's fine. I implore you to take what does and use it as a guide toward your next phase of growth. Thank you for reading this in any capacity and I wish you well.

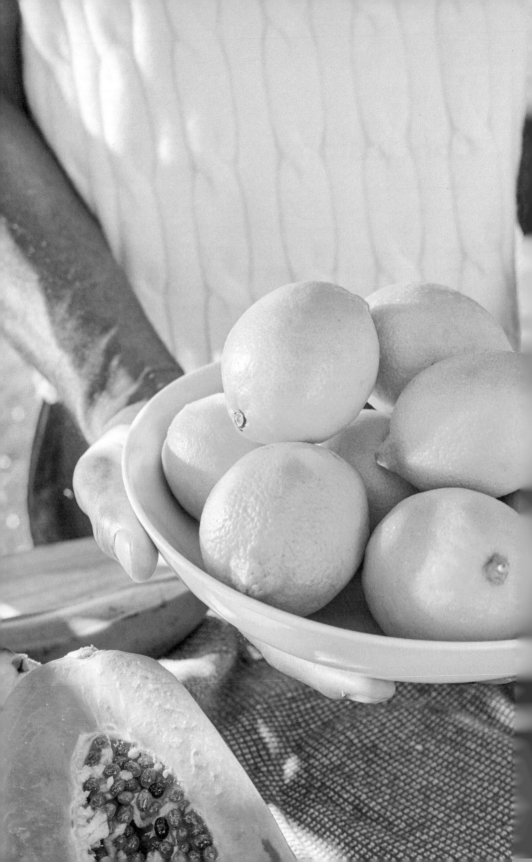